"I have known Dr. Raiszadeh well since college. He has undergone some of the best surgical training, and, having operated with him personally, I can attest to his surgical acumen with even very complex cases. What is especially unique is his long-term focus on non-operative treatment and the judicious use of surgery. I personally have seen the strong mind-body connection with spinal disorders. Also, being a big proponent of meditation and appropriate strengthening and stretching, I am confident that the reader will greatly benefit from Dr. Raiszadeh's insight and experience."

—Noman Q. Khan, MD, Fellowship-Trained Orthopedic Spine Surgeon, Board of Directors, Palo Alto Medical Foundation, 2010-2016

"We are in the midst of a devastating opioid addiction crisis, an epidemic fueled by our collective societal delusion that our lifestyle choices don't matter, that there's a quick surgical or pharmaceutical fix for everything, and that our minds have nothing to do with our physical bodies or overall health. I would have thought that the last person to help light the way out would be a spine surgeon, a specialist who is expert at doing things *to* people but not always *for* people. Which is why Dr. Raiszadeh's book is so amazing. With a deep humility, Dr. Raiszadeh uses personal stories drawn from his career and life to show us that we can heal when we focus on the root causes of our suffering, with compassion, patience, and wisdom. A must-read for anyone suffering with or treating chronic pain."

—Zubin Damania, MD, Founder, Turntable Health, ZDoggMD

"In surgery they say that 'a chance to cut is a chance to cure.' For Dr. Raiszadeh, however, the chance to *intervene* is the moment to step back and offer a holistic set of physical therapy, counseling, and lifestyle services, leaving surgery only as the last resort. *Take Back Control* offers sensible advice—backed by scientific literature and examples from Dr. Raiszadeh's clinical experience—to patients suffering from severe back pain who might be rushing toward a surgical 'solution' even though safer and cheaper options are available.

"Dr. Raiszadeh exhorts the patient to take control of his health through lifestyle changes, supported by medical care only when needed. He exhorts his surgical colleagues to remain humble in the face of the limitations and risks inherent in their skills. And in regard to the healthcare system, he shows how the transition of spine care from 'surgery first' to 'surgery when needed' can save money for society and improve well-being for patients."

—James Robinson, PhD, Leonard D. Schaeffer Professor of Health Economics, Director, Berkeley Center for Health Technology, School of Public Health, University of California, Berkeley

"Dr. Raiszadeh brings real meaning to the concept of 'person-centered care.' The optimal resolution of complex issues like back pain and function ultimately flows from support and care that empowers the individual to heal. Our challenges with opioid control and the excessive use of imaging and surgical intervention could be tempered with this physician's thoughtful approach."

—David Sayen, Former CMS Regional Administrator, Regional Administrator, U.S. Department of Health and Human Services

"Knowing what I know now, I wish I had taken Dr. Raiszadeh's advice and exhausted all options with rehab rather than going through with back surgery. There's too much that can go wrong when you expose your spinal canal to surgery. Rehab may take time, but in the long run it's a much better choice."

—Steve Kerr, Head Coach, Golden State Warriors of the NBA

"Anyone involved in the treatment of chronic musculoskeletal pain will find Dr. Raiszadeh's book to be a great resource. As the chief of orthopedics, I recommend the comprehensive approach and practices outlined in *Take Back Control* to my patients. Healthcare across the country is shifting from volume to value in order to better align the extraordinary amount spent with improved long-term outcomes. This book will help healthcare systems value a multi-disciplinary focused care team that gets patients back to an active, pain-free lifestyle without surgery. It will also help patients navigate an often complex and confusing system. On a personal note, I had a lumbar disc herniation with significant neuropathy last year. By following Dr. Raiszadeh's protocol and advice, I was able to return to hiking and mountaineering within eight months."

—Iqbal Anwar, MD, Chief of Orthopedic Surgery, Kaiser Permanente West Los Angeles Medical Center

"Struggling with back pain or sciatica is tough for anyone, but I didn't expect to be suffering from it as a retired professional athlete. After my surgery for a large disc herniation at age 42, I was determined to strengthen my back in the best way possible. My initial testing with SpineZone showed a significant weakness of my core muscles compared to the expected norm for my age. However, after completing the program, my strength has skyrocketed to the top of the charts and my back feels better than it ever has. I'm so grateful for the SpineZone program. My only regret is not having started it sooner."

—Mark Loretta, Professional Baseball Player, Retired in 2009 After a 15-Year Career as a Major League Baseball Infielder

TAKE
BACK
CONTROL

A Surgeon's Guide to Healing Your Spine Without Medications or Surgery

Kamshad Raiszadeh, MD

Published by:
OptiFit Publishers
2301 South Melrose Drive
Vista, CA 92081
Phone: 844-316-7979

ISBN: 978-0-9975918-0-4

Library of Congress Control Number: 2016909322

Medical illustrations by John and James Alesi

The stories in this book are true. However, names and identifying details have been changed to protect the privacy of all concerned.

This book is not intended to be a substitute for professional medical advice, diagnosis, or treatment. Always seek the advice of your physician or other qualified health provider with any questions you may have regarding a medical condition. Never disregard professional medical advice or delay in seeking it because of something you have read in this book.

Printed in the United States of America

This book is dedicated to all of those who feel helplessly imprisoned by spine-related pain. May you transform this pain and helplessness into insight and self-empowerment.

TABLE OF CONTENTS

FOREWORD

In 2010, Sharp Community Medical Group began a journey to better manage back and neck pain. Our goal was to create better clinical outcomes for patients, while also lowering the total cost of care for both our patients and our organization.

Over the previous few years we had heard great things about Kamshad Raiszadeh, MD, and his multi-specialty clinic, which has grown into the SpineZone of today. Dr. Raiszadeh was gaining notoriety for treating chronic back pain patients with a series of medically supervised core-strengthening exercises his team had developed, along with psychological counseling, self-empowerment training, and social support.

His emphasis on natural, minimally invasive treatment of pain relief—while certainly unconventional for a classically trained spine surgeon—was yielding great success. Not only were many of his patients able to avoid spine surgery, they also reduced or eliminated their use of prescription pills.

And so it was quickly decided that Dr. Raiszadeh and his team would become an integral part of our strategy for treating patients who suffered from chronic and debilitating pain. In many ways, this book shares what we all learned together during that journey and continue to learn today.

I am gratified that these best practices are now finding an even wider audience. You are holding in your hands a road map that can lead you out of pain, guide you to build a stronger back without surgery and potentially addictive opioids, and help you hardwire lifestyle habits that will help keep you healthy in the long run. As CEO of a large medical group with 950 physicians in San Diego—and as a physician myself—I can assure you that Dr. Raiszadeh's approach works.

Take Back Control is the compelling story of a surgeon's shift from a "specialty-driven approach"—i.e., surgery and other invasive procedures—to a "comprehensive, patient-centered diagnosis and treatment plan" where each individual is empowered to take charge of their care. And, ironically, it is offered and coordinated by the very specialist who would normally be driven by healthcare economics (known as "fee-for-service") to do *more* surgeries and *more* procedures to increase income.

In fact, what is particularly striking about Dr. Raiszadeh is how dedicated he is to helping his patients. He considers each treatment approach very carefully and subscribes quite seriously to the physician's credo to "do no harm" with his holistic approach and by always asking himself, *Is what I'm doing really helping this individual?* Dr. Raiszadeh is committed to engaging and empowering patients...and ultimately being part of the solution.

As a physician and as a healthcare executive myself, I am laser focused on two aspects of caring for patients with back and neck pain. The first, and most important, is ensuring that we deliver the very best clinical outcomes and experience for patients. We want to help them fully understand the causes of their pain, how to remedy it, and ensure that they take appropriate action, even when they sometimes face an extremely debilitating condition.

My second focus is on ensuring that the care we provide at Sharp Community Medical Group is affordable for patients. My goal is to maximize the outcome while minimizing the cost—a goal, I should mention, that is aligned with how U.S. healthcare is transforming itself today to make healthcare more affordable. In *Take Back Control,* you will read about an approach to back pain that is exceeding expectations on both fronts.

Regarding affordability, we have learned some critical lessons over the years at Sharp Community Medical Group. Back in 2010, our group cared for approximately 120,000 patients. Because our model of care included taking on the financial risk for this group, we were responsible for the overall care and affordability of services that we provided.

When we analyzed the types of services and care we provided to this group for back and neck pain over a one-year period, we learned that 12,000 patients had received some type of diagnosis and treatment. Our cost to treat them was close to $14 million...and more than 50 percent of that cost was due to things like high-cost surgical procedures, hospital and ER admissions, invasive pain management injections, expensive scanning (e.g., MRIs and CT scans), and high-cost pharmaceutical and pain management prescriptions and programs. I would venture to say, and certainly from the patient's perspective, that these were also the very kinds of medical and surgical treatments that most individuals would prefer to avoid, if at all possible.

This then is what precipitated our collaboration with Dr. Raiszadeh and his team at the first SpineZone clinic: our goal to provide patients better, more comprehensive solutions for relieving pain long-term, while also reducing the need for expensive and invasive procedures. As a result, we enrolled more than 1,400 patients in a SpineZone pilot program between 2011 and 2013.

The results? Our patients experienced exceptional gains in strength, flexibility, improvement in activity level, and relief of pain. They shared their success stories with us through many letters of support for the program. We were also able to reduce the costs of treating these patients by 25 percent year over year. (If we extrapolated that savings to our 12,000 patients over those years—assuming each of them had required treatment for back and neck pain—it would equate to a total two-year savings of $7 million.)

While patients who fully participated in and engaged in the conservative self-help program that is outlined in this book experienced remarkable and long-lasting results and improvement in their back and neck pain, they also took responsibility for their own success. To maintain such gains, you as a patient will need to commit to persistent and long-term core muscle strengthening and back hygiene with appropriate bending, lifting, and proper use of back and neck muscles in all activities.

What we found was incredibly heartening: When thoroughly educated on how the back works and given the right tools for strengthening it, patients thrived. For the most part, they enthusiastically took ownership of their physical and emotional well-being and steadily began to improve. In many cases their entire outlook on life changed for the better. If you are currently suffering from chronic back pain, I hope that you will have a similar experience.

Just like most things that are worthwhile, your recovery from pain will require your fortitude, positive attitude, and the cultivation of new habits to be successful over time and remain free from pain. But, rest assured, the wisdom, professional advice, and tools within these pages have helped thousands of patients just like you to regain an active and healthy life without pain.

I urge you then to accept the challenge to *Take Back Control.* Best wishes for a healthy, happy future.

John Jenrette, MD
Chief Executive Officer
Sharp Community Medical Group
San Diego, CA

PREFACE

I was lying on my back in the operating room, my legs completely numb and medically paralyzed. A haze engulfed me, induced by the medication that was slowly dripping into my vein. The rhythmic beeps of the heart rate monitor crashed on the shore of my consciousness, reminding me to be responsive to my situation but, at the same time, also lulling me into submission.

I glanced at the monitor that was hooked up to the scope inside my knee and I wondered why the rotating instrument with sharp teeth was aggressively trying to remove and smooth out the cartilage there. There were some mild irregularities on the surface of the cartilage, but not in areas that were causing me pain.

Then I flashed back to why I was here. I found myself wondering: Why did I make this decision to undergo surgery? Had I truly exhausted all of my other options? Did my surgeon understand the physical demands of my life and my expectations from surgery? Did I choose the right procedure for my specific life situation? In fact, did I make the choice at all...or was it somehow made for me, *not by another person but by an entire flawed system that pulls patients toward surgery like a rudderless boat that gets passively drawn by the current.*

The truth was, I felt just as disempowered in my decision to undergo surgery as I felt lying there, helplessly observing the blade slice away at my knee's cartilage...and I was an orthopedic surgeon!

Fast forwarding to the present, I am still an orthopedic surgeon, one subspecializing in spine surgery. I have found that spine surgery poses even more challenges in properly selecting candidates for elective surgery than other areas of orthopedic surgery. I see how similar my own predicament and decision-making challenges were compared to the many desperate spine patients I have treated. Yet the alluring prospect of a "quick fix" in a physically compromised and mentally distressed patient brings with it the risk of less than desirable results.

Here is the flawed cycle that I see playing out over and over again:

Patients, who are physically compromised and mentally distressed, demand to have a "quick fix" and seek out surgery. What's more, they are often addicted to the pain medications they take to dull their ongoing discomfort.

Surgeons, who have been through years of training and have skills that under the right circumstance can be very useful to patients, are often eager to cut in an attempt to cure. Most hospitals—which often get more payment when more care is provided and, subsequently, more money spent—are not incentivized to contain cost.

However, some at-risk insurance companies, medical groups, and workers' compensation, with an eye on cost containment, deny access to surgery. Patients see this as care that is being withheld from them, and therefore fight the surgery denial hoping the insurance companies will grant them their surgeries.

Primary care doctors know the right thing is to slow the drumbeat of intervention. Yet they are often not provided viable alternatives and do not have the time to teach natural ways to facilitate healing in such a complex condition. So instead, they often feel compelled to help patients to cope with pain without surgery or injections—often prescribing pain medication to at least address the symptoms.

Meanwhile, there is a nationwide trend toward a more integrative, holistic approach to healthcare with a focus on prevention. Searching for alternatives, back and neck pain sufferers are often willing to pay out of pocket for treatments such as chiropractic, massage, acupuncture, and fistfuls of supplements and holistic cures. Unfortunately, the vast majority of these treatments are not coordinated with other treatments that are covered under traditional insurance.

This leads me to the predicament I have witnessed thousands of times. I am faced with a patient who has seen their primary physician, tried some medications, undergone multiple courses of physical therapy, and even attempted injections. They have paid for holistic methods, sometimes over the course of many years, without lasting relief.

Often this patient may have a non-descript MRI abnormality and almost begs to have surgery to fix it. When I inform them that the MRI finding is actually not that bad—and that in the absence of any weakness or numbness, surgery should be avoided—they often reply with the retort: "I have tried everything else to stop the pain and nothing works."

At this point, I have no way to objectively evaluate whether the patient has done all they could to maximize their own body's healing capacity. Despite asking multiple questions, I am frustrated in not knowing whether their therapy was truly adequate. Because I have only limited exposure to the patient, it is hard to know if their expectations are realistic or if their efforts in non-operative treatment have been adequate.

Similar to many surgeons, I often make the decision to turn the patient away from surgery. If I am in private practice, this is a bad short-term business decision, given the 50 to 100 times larger financial incentive to operate versus suggesting alternative treatments. Plus, it's a lot more stressful and time consuming to try to convince the patient to forgo surgery than to just succumb to their will and go ahead with it. If I am a salaried surgeon in a large medical group or managed care organization such as Kaiser, I am likely to view this type of patient as a non-surgical burden who doesn't fall into my favored skill set.

For all of these reasons, and because of the recent changes in healthcare, I feel compelled to write this book now. In addition to making insurance coverage more accessible for low- and middle-income families, the Affordable Care Act (ACA) also supports Accountable Care Organizations that reward quality and efficiency of care rather than reimbursing based only on the quantity of care. The solutions I suggest in this book fall right in line with this "quality vs. quantity" trend.

Unfortunately, there is also a big flaw in the ACA. While most health plans must now cover preventive services such as shots, smoking cessation, and cancer screenings at no cost to the consumer (no co-pay), there has been no consensus on covered services for the prevention or for the appropriate timing of spinal injections and surgery. It is my hope that this will change in the future—and I hope my book will add to the national discussion that leads to this change.

While this book is written directly to patients, I hope it will also find its way into the hands of industry leaders and practitioners.

For healthcare administrators and policy makers, I hope that the real-world experiences and proven solutions that I share in these pages will help guide an evolution to greater integrated care solutions for the many patients who still suffer needlessly from back pain today.

For those of you who treat patients—including primary care physicians, chiropractic providers, acupuncturists, mental health professionals, and even surgeons—my hope is that this book will serve as a starting point, a source you can refer patients to, so they can learn about their spine and their body's powerful recuperative ability.

Most importantly, my goal in this book is to urge patients themselves to take back control of their spine health. I have endeavored to provide the perspective and knowledge they need to make the best, most informed decision regarding their treatment, wherever they live and whoever has treated them.

Patients, I don't want you to feel backed into a corner and rushed into a surgical decision without first understanding the power of your body's ability to heal itself. I hope my book will help you understand that power and learn how to fully access it as you move toward a healthier, happier future.

ACKNOWLEDGMENTS

I owe a debt of gratitude to the many who helped inspire this book and enable it to be born.

During the busiest times of my surgical practice, Vert Mooney, MD, provided perspective for me to expand my scope from a surgeon dealing with a condition to a practitioner addressing all aspects of a disease. His influence planted the seed that allowed SpineZone to quickly germinate and take root inside the industry.

Both my surgical and nonsurgical patients have taught me an enormous amount. They have contributed to my "aha" moment that surgery is rarely the answer for back pain, and through their feedback over the past decade have helped mold a better way for future patients.

Tim Kearin, with his 50-year history in the fitness industry, has been very helpful throughout SpineZone's decade-long development of strengthening protocols.

John Jenrette, MD, in his unwavering commitment to patients in general and to members of his physician group specifically, believed enough in what we were doing to collaborate with us in this venture, thereby helping us bring new solutions for back pain to thousands of patients in our early days.

Transforming an industry from within takes extraordinary group effort, which was made possible by Pam Erickson and my surgical practice staff and colleagues. Without their spiritual guidance, ability to reduce the pressure from my surgical practice, and understanding of my focus on the mission, this book would not have been possible.

Thanks also to the SpineZone staff, past and present: Lissa Taitano and Nick Polis, for never being too busy for the next task, for adding great insight in implementing our strengthening, stretching, posture, and nutrition protocols, and for keeping an open mind; and Frank Grant and Neil Sethi, for engaging themselves wholeheartedly in the mission of our organization. I am grateful to each of you for powering the process.

My brother, Kian Raiszadeh, MD, has brought extraordinary insight and energy to this undertaking. His commitment to leave the conventional surgeon's path has allowed us to expand our vision of what is both possible and achievable.

As a first-time book writer, I appreciate Chris Román for her patience with me and my endless edits. Thanks also to DeHart & Company Public Relations. By providing their perspective, experience, and incredible skill, Dottie DeHart and Anna Campbell have taught me how to convey my thoughts in more compelling ways.

I also relied on my wife, Shirin Raiszadeh, to improve readability, by helping me simplify medical language. Her faith in me and my unconventional career path were essential to completing this book.

And last but not least, I want to wholeheartedly thank my children as well as my extended family and all the friends who encouraged me and rallied around my singular focus on this mission.

INTRODUCTION

If you are reading this book, chances are you are suffering from significant back problems. What you might not realize is just how much company you have. Did you know that 80 percent of people will experience significant low back pain at some point during their lifetime?[1] It's true. What's more, 10-20 percent of these people are at risk for developing chronic low back pain and disability—often leading them to quit working and draw workers' compensation funds or disability benefits from the government.[2]

Even scarier, if these symptoms are not addressed in an injured worker, there is only a 50 percent chance that they will return to work after a six-month absence; this declines to a 25 percent chance following a one-year absence and is further reduced to a 1 percent chance after a two-year absence.[3, 4]

It's these chronic back and neck pain patients who account for a significant increase in health costs, about 60 percent higher than for those without back pain.[5] In a recent study published by the Bone and Joint Initiative, total direct costs for persons with a spine condition were $253 billion in 2009 to 2011, a rise of 91 percent from the $132.4 billion in 1996 to 1998, in 2011 dollars.[6] Direct costs are for those services that insurance would pay, such as for doctor visits, hospital costs, physical therapy, injections, and surgeries. This adds up to a staggering direct cost of $8,100 per back pain patient per year.[7]

In addition, an estimated 290 million work days are lost every year in the United States because of low back pain.[8] When the indirect cost of lost productivity is added to the direct cost of care, the total cost due to back pain is estimated at $560 to $635 billion per year in 2010 dollars.[9] This is greater than the annual cost of heart disease ($309 billion), cancer ($243 billion), and diabetes ($188 billion).[10]

And these numbers don't even take into account what happens when people become addicted to the opioid medications that are so frequently prescribed for back pain.

It's estimated that somewhere between 26.4 million and 36 million people worldwide abuse opioids.[11] Plus, a recent NBCNews.com article pointed out that, according to the Centers for Disease Control and Prevention, more than 47,000 people died from opioid overdoses in 2014.[12]

The good news is that, even as I put the finishing touches on this book, the CDC has recently released national standards aimed at putting a dent in the painkiller addiction problem.[13] Essentially, these guidelines suggest physicians point patients toward other methods, like therapeutic exercise, over-the-counter drugs, ice, or talk therapy, before reaching for the prescription pad. And if it turns out an opioid *is* the right choice, the CDC recommends the lowest possible dose for the shortest possible duration.

I truly believe these CDC painkiller guidelines represent a huge step in the right direction. Yet they address only part of the problem. Clearly, back pain is enormously costly, in terms of both finances and personal suffering. With so much at stake for so many, it is critical for us to develop a consistently effective solution for treating the source of pain while containing costs.

Unfortunately, there is no "easy" solution, because no two people are alike. The host of factors that make each person's condition a unique crisis requires and demands an individualized approach to healing.

To illustrate just how complicated a single patient's case can be, meet one of my patients, Dave R.

Early in my practice as a spine surgeon, back in the late 1990s, I treated Dave, a young man in his mid-20s who had suffered an on-the-job back injury as an electrician at a shipyard in San Diego. He was athletic and physically fit—very muscular, built like a bull—but in a tremendous amount of pain.

When I first met him, he had been fighting through the workers' compensation system for two years. In his quest to get people to listen to him and believe he was truly injured, he went from doctor to doctor to seek a cure for his back pain. As Dave's advocate in navigating the workers' comp system, his attorney worked tirelessly to point out to both him and others how poorly he was doing.

During that time, Dave had seen a number of pain management specialists who were all too happy to continue increasing the amount of narcotics he was taking. By the time we connected, he was on the highest possible dose of Percocet and it wasn't enough. He was desperate to get rid of the pain—he felt he couldn't work or do many other activities—and he wanted to have surgery.

When I reviewed his MRI, his spine looked normal, except for the presence of a "dark disc" in his lower back. While a dark disc is technically not completely normal, it also does not necessarily indicate a structural problem requiring surgery. It's not a fracture, a collapse, or a cause for instability of the spine. It's dark because it has lost some water content. However, the vast majority of people who have dark discs experience absolutely no pain.

In those days, spine surgeons were starting to operate on patients with chronic pain who had isolated dark discs, but my own training had led me to approach them more conservatively. In over 450 surgeries during my fellowship, we had never operated on a dark disc. So at first I discouraged Dave from surgery.

Over the course of treatment, I got to know him pretty well. Dave was a likeable, bright, engaging young man. Yet at times he seemed "out of it" from the medication. He expressed anger about his back pain, his physical limitations, and the fact that his employer and coworkers didn't believe his injury was valid.

One day I said to him, "You're not that happy guy I've seen before...and you seem very distant at times. What's going on?" He explained that he was unhappy being home on disability, but didn't feel that he could work. He also felt overwhelmed being a single dad. In short, he was in a bad place. I was very concerned that his long-term use of the medication wasn't serving him and might actually be causing an increased sensitivity to pain.

I sent him back to pain management counseling with instructions to develop a gradual weaning schedule, but he returned to me on even more medication and insisted he couldn't cope without it. I also referred him to a psychologist to help him address the anger and stress he'd expressed, but he wasn't receptive and it didn't work either. Noticing that his back muscles were continuing to atrophy, I urged him to begin some strengthening exercises to stabilize muscles in his back, but he said he was just in too much pain. He was quick to remind me that he had already undergone four different courses of physical therapy and didn't feel that they did much to build up the strength of his back.

Dave finally said to me, "I'm a young guy and normally I can lift a mountain. I can't go through the rest of my life in this amount of pain. I feel like everyone is playing games with me and that you don't think my pain is real. I feel like the whole medical system is designed to withhold care from me. You've got to fix it somehow."

We agreed that he had exhausted all the alternatives to surgery and we would proceed with a disc surgery to fuse the dark disc. Post-operatively, Dave was initially ecstatic. And, six months later, his spine looked very stable; the dark disc was fully fused. Structurally, the operation was a success. The supposed pain generator was gone.

While he was still on pain medications, he said he felt great. So when it was time for his final visit, I congratulated myself on a job well done and told myself I should have operated sooner and not doubted the dark disc as his cause of pain in the first place.

Unfortunately, Dave's long-term follow-up was not so rosy. One year after surgery, Dave was still not back to gainful employment and was angry that his workers' compensation settlement did not adequately compensate him for his pain and loss of function. When I next saw him for a follow-up, his eyes were glazed over and he seemed drugged. But as we again tried to wean him off the medication, he had increasing difficulty with pain. He insisted he needed the medication, and we agreed that there was nothing else I could do for him.

I wondered: *Could it be that initially after surgery, he experienced a placebo effect?* This can be common in surgical patients. Patients truly want to believe they are better after they've made the decision to undergo a procedure. Or: *Did I actually fix the problem but he didn't want to acknowledge this in case he decided to appeal his workers' comp case?* Or: *Could it be that his chronic narcotic dependency—and the lower pain tolerance that resulted—was the real problem?* Or, even more disturbingly: *Should I have never operated on him in the first place since it seemed like we were back to where we started?*

After that, I didn't hear from him for many years. And then, out of the blue, he sent me a letter that surprised me:

"Doc," he wrote, "I know you did everything you could for me. I'm so thankful you were willing to do the surgery. You counseled me to increase my strength, try to return to work, and get off the medication, but I wouldn't do it. I'm writing to let you know you were completely right. I was scared to return to working out. And, as a result, I became increasingly weaker. The medications were zoning me out, but I was still feeling so much pain that I became a very negative and unhappy person who was not present in my own life.

"As a result of these factors, I ruined lots of relationships…with the mother of my son and other women in my life. I couldn't hold down a job. Finally, my life got so bad that I had to dig really deep. I decided to do what you told me. I returned to the gym. You said I had to be strict with myself no matter how I felt while weaning off the medications…that I had to tell myself that my increasing pain was due to the hypersensitivity caused by the meds and not my actual pain. So I did it. And you know what? After I was done, I didn't need it anymore.

"Pain is not holding me back in my life anymore. Remember how I was such a workout king? Well, I realized I was just a shadow of myself and needed to get back to weightlifting and building muscle. I started biking and added in some other aerobic activity. I got so much energy back. I got strong again. In fact, my pain level is very low now and doesn't rule my life. I'm active and I enjoy my life. I even did some vocational retraining and am a carpenter these days...and I have a great relationship with a special woman in my life.

"So I just want to thank you for spending so much time with me. I wonder sometimes what would have happened had I listened to you sooner, even before the surgery. Better late than never, right? You know that happy guy you said you missed? He's BACK!"

Depending on which point in time you evaluate Dave's case, you would have come up with a different conclusion as to the effectiveness of certain treatments. At some points, it seemed that surgery was a fix. At others, it seemed as though medications were a fix. During certain periods of time, Dave was a victim, and during others he was empowered. Early on, it would have seemed that X-rays or MRIs alone were enough to effectively diagnose and direct treatment for his back problem. Later it became clear how complex chronic back pain can be.

I've seen this pattern of uncertainty and continual change play out over and over again throughout my 19 years in practice. And I've come to realize that this is the crucial takeaway: It is the long-term outcome of the patient that matters most. The story behind the pain—the actual person experiencing, interpreting, and even creating it—is so important.

In Dave's case, he was a fit and strong young man at the time of his injury. He became overwhelmed by his pain and negative thoughts, and was convinced that he had neither the tools nor the power to change his condition. He felt that he had to actively fight for a surgical fix. He lacked the understanding of his condition as well as the maturity, emotional support, life circumstances, or resources to choose strengthening over pain medication for a comprehensive approach to recovery. But every patient's life circumstances are completely different, and, therefore, so is their path to recovery.

What is needed is a customized and holistic approach to the problem that fits each individual. But it can be challenging for a single patient to get consistent guidance about the best treatment from a spine surgeon, a chiropractor, and a physical therapist...not to mention an insurance company, an attorney, and an employer.

How Did We Get to This Point?

Before we can talk solutions to the epidemic of chronic back pain (and all of the factors involved in treating it), we need to understand how we got here. Why *are* there so many "Daves" out there? Why are so many people in constant pain, addicted to pills, and convinced that invasive surgery is a cure-all for a problem that, in reality, *doesn't* usually require a step as drastic as going under the knife? And how has "the system" accelerated the problem?

Let's start at the beginning. In the old days, patients frequented their family doctor. If you were a patient, say 50 years ago, not only did your family doctor know you, but he knew and had likely treated your other family members as well. Therefore, he had some context to any diseases you might have suffered from. There was no insurance back then either, so you always paid "out of pocket." The doctor didn't order unnecessary tests since he knew you personally and wanted to balance your health needs and your financial ones.

It's worth mentioning here that costs were much lower in years past. (This is partially because many expensive high-tech innovations hadn't yet occurred but also because of many other factors like the lack of widespread health insurance usage and the lack of government involvement.) Still, the patients of yesterday thought twice before utilizing healthcare services since it always cost them directly. There was also likely less of a belief that we should rely on technology to understand and cure any of our discomfort. In general, the spirit of healthcare was less of an entitlement and more of a privilege, with an element of personal accountability and choice.

Eventually, though, insurance companies *did* get involved in the system. Even though accident insurance was first offered in 1850, programs like this did not evolve into the modern health insurance structure until the middle to late 20th century. Before 1965, only half of all seniors had healthcare coverage, and since they utilized the services more frequently, they paid three times as much as younger adults despite having lower incomes. (Clearly, the system has never been totally perfect or "fair.")

Government began to exert more control when the Medicare and Medicaid programs were signed into law in 1965, allowing coverage for the elderly and the poor. Medicare was later expanded to encompass patients with disabilities. Although a vital coverage, Medicare's financial difficulties are well known as more of us live longer and unmanaged access to Medicare has led to overutilization in many areas. Because of this, and for many other reasons, costs have since skyrocketed. Costs have risen despite a persistent lack of insurance coverage among many working Americans and despite the fact that many doctors are more limited in how and what they can prescribe to their patients.

Today, insurance companies—which are focused mainly on reducing costs and not as heavily incentivized to improve care—often employ "review physicians" to deny access to surgery, which only further fuels the patients' motivation to pursue it. Even though they do cover obesity screening, they often do not reimburse for instruction in physical exercise, either in a class setting or from an exercise therapist. Often these programs are too little, too late.

For its part, Medicare pays lip service to the benefits of exercise, strengthening, and non-operative care in the treatment of back pain, but its policies do not support its stated philosophy. Medicare limits the amount of therapy it allows per year and reimburses only physical therapists to perform non-operative care. Lacking the choice to visit exercise physiologists and kinesiologists, or even to attend physician-supervised programs, these patients exhaust their coverage without achieving a sustainable change in their habits.

This means those who truly need guidance, support, and monitoring must seek out their own treatments and pay out of pocket. Many elderly people with fixed incomes are not willing (or able) to make this investment, which leads to worsening cardiovascular and musculo-skeletal health.

As for injectionists and surgeons, Medicare reimburses them in a fee-for-service fashion. While this does allow providers to proceed with injections or surgery without authorization, it does not hold them accountable for the patient's overall outcome. This encourages more utilization of services and less coordination of care, since care is provided in disconnected silos.

Meanwhile, as the insurance system was evolving, the medical field was developing the most technologically advanced treatments in the world. The pharmaceutical and medical device companies brought about great innovation, revolutionizing the diagnosis and surgical treatment of all conditions, including those of the spine.

With the development of advanced diagnostic tools, we doctors were supposed to be able to pinpoint exactly what was wrong with our patients. Unfortunately, this did not happen in every case. With regard to the spine, the most relied-upon test, the MRI, is notoriously unreliable. It can show "abnormalities" in completely asymptomatic patients. Likewise, neck- and back-pain patients tend to blame their discomfort —which may actually be due to their anxieties and stresses or lack of conditioning—on their "objective" yet completely irrelevant MRI findings.

Motivated by the belief that every pain has a scientifically identifiable cause, many patients expect modern medicine to "fix it." And often, we can. With the help of innovative surgeons, the medical device industry has enabled us to repair spinal fractures, remove tumors, straighten and realign deformities of the spine, remove compression on nerves, and treat spinal infections. We have used similar technology to try to remove the most common presumed source of pain, the disc. But as we will discover in the following pages, the source of back and neck pain is not always so simple to identify and fix.

As the medical industry has surged ahead, patients have become more sedentary than ever before. Not only do we take cars to our destination instead of walking, we often sit all day at work. What's more, we are too busy keeping up with frantic schedules to exercise regularly. Ironically, despite fueling the great advances that have revolutionized our work, home, and social lives, technology has not only left the back problem unsolved, it has contributed to it. With our minds occupied and entranced, we often stay buried in or contorted around our laptops, mobile phones, game consoles, or desktops, compromising the structures in our spines.

Our diets have also changed for the worse. Processed foods have become widely available and inexpensive. We subsist on packaged "non-foods" in lieu of the real nourishing foods that have sustained humanity for thousands of years. Additives such as high fructose corn syrup taste great, but only whet our appetite to eat more, feel less satiated, and signal our bodies to store more fat on our frames. Between our now overweight and unconditioned bodies, our constant imprisonment in poor posture, and our ever-increasing stress levels (which as we will soon learn also impact the problem), it is no coincidence that everyone has started developing chronic back pain.

The Healthcare Practitioner's Current Reality

Today, I recognize that I did not have the resources or capability to evaluate whether Dave's non-operative treatment was adequate. This is a problem that all spine surgeons face, to a degree. Even though we all refer patients for non-operative treatment—mainly having them undergo physical therapy—there's no accepted standard to tell us, "Okay, our non-operative efforts have failed and it's time to resort to surgery."

The challenge is that the physical therapists, chiropractors, and medical doctors who serve as the first lines of defense often evaluate and treat spinal condition patients very differently from one another. You don't need an advanced degree to know that patients won't get consistent results if disparate practitioners all speak different languages and treat patients with dissimilar diagnoses and plans. Plus, they tend to employ passive modalities that focus mainly on reducing pain complaints and don't empower patients to treat themselves.

Meanwhile, pain management physicians have a large arsenal of strong medications and prescribe them more liberally than do other practitioners. They often focus on the patient's pain level and not on her functional level. The injections they prescribe often temporarily work but are not proven to have any long-term effectiveness.

Finally, consider the surgeons. Because typically there is no integrated approach to help different kinds of care providers to work together to assess and develop a treatment plan, we spinal surgeons often find ourselves in the position of being the patient's "last resort." And because our training focuses on fixing what is broken—and is often very isolated from other types of care providers and treatment modalities—we end up with lots of patients like Dave.

In other words, desperate patients who have seemingly "failed" to improve by all other modalities come to spinal surgeons for a fix—and we often oblige with (not surprisingly) a surgical solution. Unfortunately, because we are not always dealing with an obvious problem with a clear-cut solution (like, for instance, a broken bone), surgical outcomes can vary greatly.

Chronic pain is now recognized as a complex "psychophysiological" behavior pattern. In other words, it's not purely a sensory phenomenon that you can easily divide into distinct psychological and physical components. And, in my experience over the years, addressing it properly requires a multi-pronged approach. Unfortunately, such an approach has not been widely available.

To fill this void in the marketplace for spine health, my team and I created a program called SpineZone. It incorporates many of the above-mentioned principles, all integrated within one coordinated and well-orchestrated system. All patients, including those with the most deconditioned core muscles, receive strengthening that they are able to tolerate even if they are suffering from pain. We record, follow, and treat their postural issues as well as provide both home exercises and stretching programs.

During therapy sessions, patients are supervised by a combination of exercise physiologists and physical therapists in order to achieve cost effective and sustainable results. The patient is guided through the entire process by a spine "coach," who is the patient's go-to person. It's the spine coach's job to coordinate treatment and navigate the patient through the process.

If a patient is focused on previous MRIs or X-rays, or is afraid to engage in rehabilitation for any reason (including previous surgeries), a physician assistant or spine surgeon reviews their concerns and places (often irrelevant) diagnostic findings in the proper context. We educate patients and reassure them that most conditions will improve without intervention—again, *despite* significant findings on an MRI.

There are, however, some cases where we become concerned by the patient's lack of progress or by certain physical examinations' findings. Only in rare cases such as these do we recommend appropriate specialized X-rays or advanced imaging such as an MRI.

In order to follow our results, we initially measure the patient's core strength and use proprietary software to monitor the improvement of this strength as well as other outcome and satisfaction measures during the course of the program. The coaches and clinic managers are alerted when there are warning signs that a patient is not progressing. This is when the team charts an updated treatment course by obtaining input from each other and expanding the care to include the skill sets of everyone on the team.

We obtain data from the insurers and medical groups to continue monitoring the participants' utilization of health services and to assess the cost-effectiveness and value of our program. We regularly report these findings back to the medical groups. Our goal is to have an integrated team employing the best available knowledge from multiple different specialties in order to provide a systematic way to treat patients—all focused on getting the best, reproducible results.

By the way: SpineZone patients often have great success in cutting back on prescription drugs of all kinds, including narcotic pain medications. (More on this in Chapter 3.)

Now, I'd like to touch on the sensitive issue of money. The reality is that your insurance may not pay for the best possible treatment as described in this book—and if you're on Medicare, without some reform, it definitely won't. But your health is absolutely worth investing in.

Here is the truth: The best treatment option for dealing with your chronic back pain likely isn't surgery or injections. It also isn't likely to be years of addictive prescription drugs or a few rounds of physical therapy either, yet these are often the go-to treatments that insurance companies are willing to pay for. The solutions to lasting relief from chronic back pain *are* likely to be the ones I will describe in this book. These treatments are life-changing for many patients—but only if they believe that a pain-free life is worth investing in. They must be willing to take the time to understand their conditions and also invest personally in any treatments that may not be covered by insurance.

You may be thinking to yourself how unfair it seems to pay monthly insurance premiums and still be expected to additionally pay for the program that actually heals you from pain. I agree, to an extent. Unfortunately, this is where we are *today*—I hope this changes soon and

I believe it will eventually, as everyone becomes more comfortable with the idea that a holistic and integrated approach to healthcare is the commonsense answer that we've been looking for.

In the interim, I encourage you to change your perception of what is "worth" paying for. Often people don't think twice about committing to expensive cable TV packages, for example, but are reluctant to spend an equivalent amount on services that may have a far greater impact on their quality of life. Also, many health plans and medical groups' experience have shown that it's better to have patients share some of the responsibility for their care so they are more vested and don't either overutilize or take the service for granted. (This is the reason for co-pays and other shared cost structures.)

You may not be struggling with Dave's addiction to pain medications or his emotional challenges, but I suspect his journey resonates with you as a fellow sufferer of chronic pain. I encourage you to remain positive and read this book with an open mind. Whether you are young or old, trying to recover from an acute injury or a structural defect you've had for a lifetime, you deserve the least invasive solution to your pain that offers the greatest hope for long-term recovery. You deserve to put the pain behind you and get your life back on track.

IT'S ALL ABOUT *YOU*

When I decided to write *Take Back Control*, my goal was to share my many decades of experience on how patients can achieve truly transformational change for back and neck pain—often without surgery and potentially addictive pain medications.

In the course of my career, I've found that I could often make a far greater impact by educating patients about the true risks and potential benefits of surgery—and giving them the confidence and information they needed to commit to less invasive alternatives—than I could by following my profession's natural bias toward cutting. This is why I founded SpineZone, the integrated care clinics here in San Diego that put all these pieces together.

As a spine surgeon with a busy clinical practice, I've been humbled over the years as I've come to fully appreciate the power of the human body's innate ability to recuperate—not just to cope and compensate, but frequently, to fully repair and correct itself—if provided the right tools and education. My experience in this respect has sometimes been at odds with my extensive professional training as a surgeon.

I've moved from a view that pain is caused by isolated and well-documented spinal disorders to a more in-depth integrated view of the delicate interplay between the muscles and bones that comprise the entire core of the body. I've also gained a great appreciation for the power of the mind-body connection.

Perhaps one of my most surprising discoveries is that good clinical outcomes depend a great deal upon the actual *individual* experiencing the pain. The truth is that we each bring experiences, habits, and a unique physiological and psychological makeup to our recovery from back pain. We will explore each of these aspects in-depth in the coming chapters so you understand what you as a patient can do to maximize your opportunity to recover given these factors.

So get ready…because your recovery doesn't likely depend on a magic pill or quick-fix surgery. Rather, *you* are the one who will determine the trajectory of your own recovery from back pain. I know that, armed with the knowledge and confidence I hope this book will inspire, you'll make the best decision for you.

CHAPTER 1

IS A CHANCE TO CUT *ALWAYS* A CHANCE TO CURE?

> "Change is the end result of all true learning."
>
> —Leo Buscaglia

I think I have always been interested in restoring function to the body. Even before I went to college or medical school, I was an athlete who played competitive soccer and tennis. I suffered a number of sports injuries in high school, including repeated ankle sprains. In fact, when I was 17, I'd injured the same ankle so many times that the orthopedic surgeon I saw finally put me in a five-week cast for a "time-out" on re-injury. It was an early wake-up call that I wish I'd heeded in the years to come.

Joints and muscles fascinated me. I was a biochemistry major at UC Berkeley, and despite a heavy load of courses, I tried out for both the tennis and soccer teams and truly enjoyed practicing with the teams my freshman year.

But that summer I tore a ligament in my knee—the anterior cruciate ligament or "ACL." (This ligament is a very tough band of tissue that connects the thigh bone to the leg bone and is vital in providing stability for sports that require quick changes of direction, such as tennis.)

While my self-image was of someone who was strong, fast, and capable, tennis was not my primary focus at school. Studying was. Even though I was continuing to play in competitive tournaments, my knee and its associated muscles were not as conditioned as my teammates' were. Tennis involves a lot of cutting...a lot of start and stop that can be hard on your knees if you don't strengthen properly. I believe this is why I sustained the injury.

I had my knee evaluated by an orthopedist who told me he could reconstruct the ACL, but I was firmly opposed to the surgery as it was performed in the early 1980s. ACL reconstruction was not as refined and routine as it is today. Since I felt that I had missed my window of opportunity to compete for a spot on the team, I resigned myself to a lower level of competition. Despite the occasional pain, I continued to play tennis the best I could. I didn't have a lot of free time so I played hard whenever I had the opportunity.

After I completed my degree at Berkeley, I was admitted to UC San Francisco, one of the top medical schools in the country. While I had breezed through high school and college at the top of my classes, the pace of learning in med school was frenetic. We had to learn in weeks what we had spent a year on in college.

The pressure to perform well in a group of other elite students was high. The first two years required massive amounts of rote memorization. We had to learn every nerve and muscle in anatomy and their function in physiology...down to the tiniest detail; to understand every intricacy of the human body, from how the heart rate is affected by breathing to how we take gasses in.

The next two years consisted of one- to three-month clinical rotations where I absorbed knowledge as fast as I could. A world-renowned physician would introduce us to a topic and would then quiz us in front of our peers on our in-depth knowledge the very next day. I spent my days seeing patients in three or four Bay Area hospitals on rotations in the emergency department, surgery service, OB/GYN, neurosurgery, internal medicine, orthopedics, family practice, and more. Then I'd hit the books in the evenings.

When I found a (rare) free moment, I'd indulge in some ultimate Frisbee, compete in a tennis tournament, or meet for soccer practice with a few of my peers (several were top-notch athletes). But I think I did more harm than good to my knee, because, again, I was trying to make up for lost time without any strength training.

Meanwhile, my dean at UC San Francisco tried to convince me to become a primary care physician rather than a surgeon. At the time, there was a great need for more primary care physicians to guide integrated treatment for patients rather than more subspecialists like surgeons. But I was uninterested in diagnosing things I couldn't fix. Clearly, my naïveté and arrogance about the role of surgery were evident in this narrow-minded view of physicians' roles. I didn't come to understand or appreciate the importance of a more integrated and holistic approach until years later.

Rather, the more I learned in medical school about what orthopedics entailed—repairing shoulders, knees, ankles, and wrists—the more it appealed to my desire

to make a meaningful difference in the lives of the patients I saw. And in the world of surgeons, an often-re-
peated saying is: "A chance to cut is a chance to cure."

A chance to cut is a chance to cure.

In other words, surgical training is based on the
premise that we are looking for things we can diagnose
and fix. This is excellent when we see patients with
clear structural deformities, tumors, or other patholog-
ical problems, but can be less so when patients have
pain complaints or more complex disorders that may
not match up with the tools in our tool box.

Residency Reinforces My Role as "Repairer"

After four years of general and elective training in
med school, I embarked on the next stage of my gradu-
ate medical training, a five-year residency in orthopedics
under the supervision of senior physician educators at
UC Davis in Sacramento, CA. This included an initial
year of a surgical internship where I worked clinically
in every surgical specialty under the close supervision
of mentors. The next few years included orthopedic
subspecialties such as hands, shoulders, trauma, sports
injuries...and I loved them all. That training confirmed
my earlier interest in fixing things so people could get
back to their lives quickly.

I experienced a deep sense of pride and satisfaction when presenting the X-rays of a challenging fracture that I fixed to a world-renowned trauma surgeon,

soaking in his accolades. I was so focused on fixing things that I didn't fully appreciate the importance of the personal stories that accompanied patients' injuries and spinal problems. At the time, their histories and the context of their injuries didn't seem relevant. It's not that I didn't care about them; it's that I thought that "fixing" their problem as efficiently as possible was my main objective.

Yet on occasion I would see a patient whose story shook this single-minded focus. I remember the case of a young woman who first came in with a suspicious story of a shoulder dislocation when "horsing around" with her boyfriend. She was admitted to the hospital one year later after being pushed by the same boyfriend off of a two-story balcony and fracturing her thigh bone, pelvis, spine, and forearms. (Could I have done more than just relocate her shoulder when I first saw her? What if I had asked more questions with caring and compassion?)

In general, though, my sole focus was on the intricate work of spine surgery. The simple elegance and functionality of the spine fascinated me. For instance, the gentle curves of the spine have functional utility in distributing the stress of gravity. Also bone, which is often regarded as such a hard and rigid structure, is actually composed of an elegant combination of spongy material that nourishes our blood and a living matrix of tough minerals that are constantly being molded by cells that are responsive to the forces of gravity. In short, the spine is a moving masterpiece.

By the third year of my orthopedic residency, I knew that I wanted to become a spine surgeon. And I was well on my way to becoming a master technician. As a surgeon in training, I honed my skill and talent for complex surgery. I acquired the skills necessary to treat multiple pathologic conditions. However, we were less focused on the patient as a unique individual with sometimes complex emotional and psychological issues than we were on the pathology that we were learning to fix. We gave little thought as to how factors other than the obvious abnormality on the MRI or X-ray influence the outcome of surgery or whether surgery was warranted at all if other factors were correctly addressed.

Doctors often choose their specialties based on a combination of their personalities and preferences. Like many other surgeons, I was lured by the amazing potential of surgery to permanently fix very disabling diseases. Unfortunately, there are only a finite number of conditions for which surgery is helpful, and the fixes are not always permanent.

The problem arises when we as surgeons try to pit our surgical skills against a condition for which it is not necessarily intended. The analogy often quoted is that "when one has a hammer, more things start to look like nails." This can create an unfortunate blind spot in many of us, because we are frequently in the position of determining whether a patient is a candidate for surgery, which is the domain where we feel most capable.

> *When one has a hammer, more things start to look like nails.*

When all of your training centers on performing surgeries, and when your livelihood depends on doing so, it's difficult to see other solutions. Yet somehow we need to shift our perspective if we are to reduce unnecessary spine surgeries and direct patients to less invasive solutions.

In the case of my knee injury, I finally elected for an ACL reconstructive surgery during my residency. Because I had a bit more time for sports than I'd had during medical school, I began to entertain thoughts about getting back to competitive tennis. I watched one of my chief residents undergo the procedure—which had now become more refined and routine—and recover well. So after consulting with a number of my orthopedic colleagues and getting their recommendations, I finally moved forward.

In hindsight, I wish one of those many orthopedic colleagues had impressed upon me the importance of strengthening and conditioning if I wanted to continue to play sports at a competitive level. The surgery did ultimately help me, as I could play tennis again after completing the standard rehabilitation. But I didn't feel as strong as I once did, so I turned to squash as my main sport, which was a little more protective of my knee and also fit my availability better than tennis tournaments.

I gradually improved in squash, playing in tournaments as high as "A" level. I water and snow skied often. However, over the next three years, I gradually started to feel an intense burning pain in the back of my knee that would occasionally keep me up at night. Since it seemed to feel better when I worked out and played, I continued to be active. Thinking that I had learned the appropriate exercises, I did not engage in a consistent, measured strengthening program. I did not seek out the best practitioners in non-operative care and subject them to the same scrutiny as my surgeon. At this point, I hadn't yet connected the dots between my level of conditioning and the longevity of my joints and my level of function.

An All-Consuming Fellowship in the Big Apple

And then I moved to New York City for fellowship training at the Hospital for Joint Diseases, where I would sub-specialize in spine surgery. I was excited about moving to the Big Apple ("If you can make it there, you can make it anywhere!") and I spent quite a bit of time walking around the city.

Due to the heavy surgical schedule and the many hours spent on my feet, there was no time for sports. The hospital was a very busy place with eight full-time spine surgeons who served as my mentors and exposed me to a diverse group of patients and pathology. It was an incredible training opportunity.

My days started early, by rounding on patients in the hospital at 5:30 a.m. so we could report their progress to the attending physician when he arrived. Then we'd head to the top floor for a quick breakfast to watch the sun rise over the gleaming Twin Towers. It was a glorious sight.

Several mornings a week, we'd operate on cases that would take 12 to 15 hours. The evenings were spent cramming to acquire more knowledge as fast as we could. Other days we'd prepare talks to teach and lecture residents there. While we were supervised closely during our residency, we were expected to operate more independently as fellows, in preparation for soon having our own surgical practices. Although I had a phenomenal surgical training experience, I did not learn much about non-operative treatment or how to deal with chronic pain patients.

However, I did learn a lot about reconstructing spines. Spine surgery involving a large deformity, such as scoliosis, typically consists of hundreds of steps. The surgeon is essentially disrupting and then rebuilding a new structure where the success of each step is dependent on the precision and attention to detail used in the step that came before. In fact, I remember one case that was done with three surgeons over the course of two days.

During my fellowship, I learned specific techniques to hold onto the vertebrae. This involved anchoring large screws into the vertebrae through the pedicle. (The pedicle is a tiny cylindrical bony structure that lies on each side of the spinal canal, within a millimeter or two of nerves or the spinal cord that have vital function.)

It's a challenging process, because the surgeon must try to thread the eye of the needle, which is the inner spongy bone of the pedicle, even though it is obscured by irregularly shaped bone. It takes vast experience to learn how to apply just the right amount of pressure at the exact location so as to drill down to the eye of the needle (middle of the pedicle) before the outer bone of the pedicle gives way to jeopardize a nerve or blood vessel. There is a sense of extreme danger as one tries to finesse this delicate process.

A similar experience occurs when spine surgeons must go through the belly of a patient to reach the front of the spine. We must move guts, vessels, and the aorta and vena cava out of the way. If you slip, or pull the retractor too hard, vessels tear as the abdomen quickly fills with blood. A small nick could cause fatal blood loss.

We also received ample opportunity to practice working near the spinal cord and nerves. These nervous tissues are bathed in spinal fluid, which is sealed in a thin sac called the "dura." When there is a disc herniation or tightness of the spinal canal caused by degeneration (stenosis), surgeons must remove the pressure while avoiding puncturing or tearing the dura. The danger is that any violation of this outer layer, which can become thinned and tethered by scarring, will result in a gush of clear cerebrospinal fluid (CSF) under pressure.

When this puncturing or tearing of the dura occurs, which is almost guaranteed to happen at some point in every spine surgeon's career, it's heart wrenching. The surgeon knows that he or she needs to suture the often crumbly and ragged edges of the dura together, even though it is a delicate structure with the consistency of thin, wet tissue paper and can be buried eight to nine inches deep into the skin.

It's critical that this tiny layer of tissue is restored enough to not allow leaking of the spinal fluid. Spinal fluid bathes the brain and spinal cord, and since it is under pressure, it can continue to leak out of the wound. If the fluid becomes infected, meningitis can result, which can be life threatening. Even with a successful repair, patients often experience severe spinal headaches.

Precision is critical as a surgeon removes scar tissue or pulls disc herniations or compressing ligaments off of the dura. In fact, many practicing spine surgeons are still uncomfortable removing extensive scar tissue surrounding the dura, even after years of training. It can take surgeons years to become comfortable working around this nemesis…this bluish tube called the dura.

Many, many hours go into the making of a master spine surgeon. Our reward is the privilege of being entrusted with our patients' bodies. Our performance must be superlative during every surgical episode, as those hours can literally transform a patient's life for better or worse.

> *Many, many hours go into the making of a master spine surgeon. Our reward is the privilege of being entrusted with our patients' bodies.*

My Knee Pain Demands a Second Surgery

On a personal note, I was so busy with my professional training during my New York fellowship that I only rarely played squash. Instead, I spent all my time on my feet in surgery—but this too took its toll. By the middle of my fellowship, my knee was more painful than ever. I was having trouble standing. And I was confused by the decline in function since I'd been playing competitive squash just a year before. How could it get so bad so fast?

I was desperate to put an end to the pain so I went for a consult with one of the physicians at our hospital—in fact this was the physician who had operated upon my mentor and lead spine surgeon. He looked at my MRI and said that while it looked good, he suspected I had some cartilage damage on the back of my knee and recommended surgery. Again, he was a surgeon, so in his mind, a chance to cut was a chance to cure.

In retrospect, I now see how my decision to proceed with surgery was impacted by my physical and mental state at the time. I kept a grueling schedule that required me to stand for prolonged periods of time as a spine surgeon in-training. With time to exercise just once a week (instead of six days a week as I used to do), I could feel my old knee injury acting up. I was too consumed by other duties to find and commit to the best rehabilitation program.

My knee had become weaker. The muscles that were usually strong and flexible were now less so…a condition that I now realize is commonly associated with an increase in knee pain. I was in a transition period of my life, exiting the roaring 20s that had been filled with athletic endeavors and entering into my 30s. This new period would be filled with career and family building, while living in New York—far from the West Coast where I had grown up and spent my formative years. I was neither physically nor mentally in an ideal condition to make the best decision.

My surgeon surely had good intentions. But his view of me as a spine surgeon who was engaged in a profession with relatively low physical demands did not correspond with my self-image as an athlete. He didn't really hear me when I explained that I wanted to get back to water skiing and squash or tennis at a competitive level. Rather, he assumed that as a spine surgeon, my life would be consumed by my work and that I would remain relatively sedentary. His goal was really just to relieve my pain while standing so I could be more comfortable at work.

For my part, I didn't have the awareness to realize that I wasn't the same person that I was in my 20s; I couldn't just jump out on the court and expect to be able to play well without training, especially given my previous knee injury. This mismatch of unrealistic expectations by both patient and surgeon didn't make for an optimal treatment decision. In fact, today, I regret that surgery, and I can only wish that I had known then what I know now.

During the surgery, I had a spinal anesthetic, so my legs were numb and immobile, yet I was awake and could watch the repair of the cartilage defect that was causing my burning pain. When I saw him aggressively trimming the cartilage under my kneecap, however, I was confused. While it's true I had consented to allow him to use his discretion on what needed to be addressed once he entered my knee, the part he was shaving—despite not totally looking normal—was not causing me any symptoms.

I am sure that if he understood I was an athlete who intended to really maximize the use of that joint, he would have acted more conservatively. And yet, even though I was familiar with the procedure, I was also the patient…and an anesthetized one at that. I felt vulnerable. So I didn't question his judgment.

Afterwards, he assured me that all would be well; the operation had been a success. A few early precautions were given, but there was no mention of specific strengthening exercises for my knee's continued conditioning. He had operated on my mentor, who could stand to perform surgeries without pain, but he had never aspired to the athleticism that I did.

My point in sharing this saga is to illustrate how I became caught up (willingly, I'll admit) in a system that promoted surgery as an instant solution to my ongoing knee problems. In short, I had morphed from a person who was absolutely opposed to surgery in college to someone who easily consented to a second surgery due to my desperate state of mind during my fellowship. How did this happen?

It's interesting to me that when we suffer an injury as a child or young adult, we have faith that our bodies will heal. And yet, somehow as we age, we lose that confidence in our natural ability to repair and often give away our power to doctors or other healthcare providers. I see this with many of my patients. I have also observed that a second surgery is easier to rationalize than a first one.

We give away our power to doctors.

My Professional Life Begins…and with It Comes an Aha! Moment

After that second surgery, my pain did improve, and I got back to enjoying squash and a more active lifestyle as I began my professional life as a spine surgeon practicing in San Diego, CA. I joined the practice of Dr. Behrooz Akbarnia, an internationally recognized and world-class deformity surgeon who continued to provide top-notch spine training to me.

Fellowship training alone is only the starting point since the first few years of practice are crucial to the development of an accomplished spinal surgeon. My work with Dr. Akbarnia built upon the early framework I'd learned during my fellowship to enable me to correct even more complex structural issues than I'd previously attempted, and to think about them in a systematic way.

I was also fortunate because Dr. Akbarnia introduced me to the "who's who" of spine surgery. One of these surgeons was Dr. Art Steffee, the physician who popularized the use of the pedicle screw (described earlier) in spine surgery. Pedicle screws are a key component in correcting any kind of spine deformity or stabilizing a fracture, and they truly revolutionized spine surgery.

I also had the opportunity to learn from Dr. Jurgen Harms, a renowned German surgeon who showed me brave, creative, and eye-opening solutions to successfully operating on the worst of the worst deformities. Dr. Stefano Boriani also visited us to share his vast experience with treating spinal tumors.

One of my most enlightening experiences was spending time with Dr. Mark Asher, a well-known deformity surgeon in Kansas, where much research on scoliosis was done. Unlike the transient populations in California and New York, patients who farmed the Midwest stayed close to home and thus provided an opportunity to study non-operative cases over a lifetime.

Many of these heavy laborers remained active and resilient into their 50s and 60s, despite X-rays taken in their adolescence that showed scoliosis severe enough to require surgery given the prevailing wisdom. I got a sense that perhaps we were over-operating, and that our patient selection and operative criteria were not fully taking into account how well patients could cope with their spinal conditions if they stayed strong and active.

Yet on the other end of the spectrum, my thinking was challenged by the emerging trend where doctors were beginning to try treating neck and low back pain through spine surgery. Suddenly, I found myself considering surgery in a patient population that we had dismissed as "non-surgical" both in training and during my first year in practice.

And then I had an "aha!" moment that would transform my approach to treating spinal conditions forever and renew my faith in the power of strengthening. I'd begun enthusiastically bicycling and swimming since I had less time for tennis tournaments as a physician in private practice, and was awed by the power of conditioning. My knee was better than ever.

I noticed that as my quadriceps strength increased with bicycling, it seemed to directly correlate with both improvement in my knee function in other sports and a decrease in the pain. The more I cycled, the more stable the joint felt. My tennis and squash games improved, to the amazement of my brother, who is an orthopedic surgeon specializing in sports injuries.

When he examined me, he couldn't reconcile the instability he noticed with the relative stability he saw when I was retrieving the tennis ball. As former captain of the Cal Berkeley tennis team, he was particularly surprised by how well I could still change direction with my unstable knee when I played. The strong stabilizing muscles around my knee compensated for the ACL deficiency.

Likewise, I noticed that when I swam, an old shoulder dislocation that I sustained from kickboxing improved through masters swimming workouts. The pain disappeared, and I got my tennis serve back. That's when the miracle of strength training really hit me.

I had always known, and it is well described in the literature, that strength training increases joint stability. (Through my own experience, I realized that this occurred to a higher degree than I would have imagined.) Yet I had also always been taught that cartilage defects and arthritis were relentlessly progressive and debilitating. Though a cartilage defect was identified during my first surgery, I realized that the symptoms related to this defect varied based on the level of my own conditioning and weren't necessarily progressive or debilitating.

By focusing on strength and flexibility, I realized, I was able to compensate for deficiencies I had in stability and alignment. So it finally hit me: Why weren't we consistently using spine strengthening to treat spine instability and arthritis?

*So it finally hit me: Why weren't we
consistently using spine strengthening
to treat spine instability and arthritis?*

When it comes to knees, research shows that even relatively minor increases in the strength of the quadriceps—the muscles that run along the front of the thigh—can help reduce the risk of knee osteoarthritis and its progression and also reduce pain.[1] One study compared three groups of patients—those with the most strength, a moderate amount of strength, and the weakest—and found that those with the most strength had only half as much chance of getting symptomatic knee osteoarthritis as the weakest third did.

The Arthritis Foundation notes that exercise can be helpful for other forms of arthritis, too, because it strengthens the muscles that support the joint.

For example, it is well documented that strengthening of the rotator cuff muscles is vital for shoulder function and stability. Proper exercise also reduces the risk of knee injury. In fact, young girls have a tendency to injure their ACL due to the alignment of their knees. Proper rebalancing has been shown to markedly reduce this risk.[2] The ankle joint is similar in responding to proper alignment.

If strengthening works to heal knees, shoulders, and ankles, why not spines? I have become more and more convinced that, in many cases, surgery isn't the right answer. But before we can adopt a less invasive approach, we must change mindsets—and that means the mindsets of patients and surgeons alike.

We Need a Shift Toward Long-Term Thinking...

To this day, I question the necessity of my second surgery. I often wonder if a physician had pointed out to me (back during my residency), that the main reason for my pain was my weekend warrior approach to competitive sports without an equal commitment to strengthening and conditioning, whether I would've made a different decision with a potentially better outcome.

I wish someone had cautioned me to step back from my desperation and encouraged me to find 30 minutes a day for bicycling or strengthening during those last six months of my fellowship to stabilize my knee for those 12- to 15-hour days of standing—and then to focus on a more sustained approach to conditioning once I completed that training and had a few more hours available in my days. I am still surprised that I didn't step back to realize this.

I needed someone to explain to me—and emphasize—that my body could most definitely "reheal," even if it couldn't grow new cartilage…that I was going to be fine after some conditioning because I just had a small defect in the cartilage in the back of my knee that I could still overcome. While I'd never have the knee of a 17-year-old again, the body is remarkable in its ability to compensate for structural problems and stress, which we will talk more about in the pages to come.

When I had the second surgery, the real problem was my state of mind. I had invested years to get to where I was and needed to learn this complex new field—spine surgery—yet I was experiencing pain standing for the many hours it required. I was in a vulnerable situation with a short-term focus. I feared the loss of my athletic abilities and had unrealistic expectations of my activity level given my other considerable commitments. Due to all of these factors, my pain tolerance was low.

I wasn't exercising enough or making time for restorative pursuits. The physical therapist took me through some exercises, but had no measure of my fitness or strength (and even if he did, he was certainly not communicating with my surgeon). Modifying my activity level didn't seem like an option at the time. My stress level was high and I wanted a quick fix.

I don't ever want my patients to make a similar decision, where their desperation leads them to seek a quick surgical solution when a less invasive option might yield an even better long-term outcome.

It's quite common for me to see patients who insist they need to at least try surgery as an option, even if it has a low likelihood of success. Early in my practice, I accepted this as a patient's consent to move forward with a procedure. These days, when I hear these sentiments expressed, it's frequently a red flag that a person is desperate and may not be well informed about all their alternatives or the consequences of their decisions.

Is a chance to cut *always* a chance to cure? After such extensive technical training (as well as what I thought was excellent knowledge of non-operative treatment options), I once thought my training was complete. I felt that I was well suited to evaluate patients, refer the ones who needed other treatments, and select the ones that I could cure surgically. Now I know differently.

…and a More Integrated Approach

While we surgeons have trained to become master technicians, we don't typically work directly with other healthcare providers as an integrated team. I know that I didn't, early in my career. I'd send patients to physical therapy for six to twelve sessions or an injection, and if the patient did not improve, I considered that a failure of non-operative treatment and the patient a likely candidate for surgery.

WHAT NEEDS TO CHANGE IN MEDICAL SCHOOL TRAINING

Learning how to treat patients more holistically must begin in medical school. This is a huge topic that my small book can't hope to adequately cover. However, just to hit the high spots, medical schools need to:

- Foster curiosity and research, especially when it comes to alternative, natural, and non-invasive treatments that show promise (even if there is no current scientific proof).
- Truly gauge any intervention against the best, non-invasive alternative. In other words, make sure any intervention is better than the best non-surgical measures we could implement (not just better than if we did nothing).
- Allow students to spend time and do rotations with holistic care providers. They should be able to receive first-hand knowledge of these other practitioners and their treatment methods.
- Teach students not to dismiss holistic treatments that show promise in improving patients' lives—yet continue to strive to scientifically evaluate every treatment.
- Help students develop a discerning and skeptical eye when evaluating science that is funded by pharmaceutical companies with vested interests.

- Spend more time educating students on preventative care.
- Do a better job of honing communication skills so they can educate patients, assuage their fears, and steer them toward more natural, less invasive alternatives when appropriate.
- Educate students regarding the healthcare system and specifically the value (cost versus impact) of each type of care.

However, my eyes were finally opened regarding other treatment options. I'm so grateful I met Dr. Vert Mooney, who materially changed my thinking. Vert was a well-known and published surgeon who was a professor of orthopedic surgery at UC San Diego.

He was previously the chairman of orthopedic surgery at the University of Texas at Austin and had decades of experience with non-operative care of the spine. He had started an innovative spinal strengthening program as part of the UC San Diego Department of Orthopaedic Surgery, employing well-tested rehabilitation machines for back pain that he'd used with great success on patients since the 1970s.

I first met Dr. Mooney after my own training. He would attend weekly conferences when I was training other surgeons at the fellowship training program I had helped found with Dr. Akbarnia. Dr. Mooney challenged me when I told him a patient had "failed non-operative treatment." "How did they 'fail' exactly?" he'd ask me. "How do you define that?" When I'd tell him they'd seen a chiropractor and a physical therapist, he'd dig deeper: "How many visits? What exactly did they do? Did they focus on strengthening the spine, and if so, how did they measure and improve the strength? How did they know they had accomplished the appropriate strength and conditioning levels?" he'd ask.

Eventually, I partnered with Vert to move his program, called "WellStrong," into my office with his machines, which was the first step toward creating the SpineZone centers that exist today in San Diego. We have now grown to multiple centers and recently logged our 50,000th patient visit.

While I'm still a full-time practicing spine surgeon—I specialize in treating deformities and back and neck pain using minimally invasive and muscle sparing surgeries—I am now finally part of a holistic, integrated treatment team. Different practitioners work together to provide the least invasive treatments and focus on helping patients develop habits that lead to long-term better function and quality of life.

With this team approach, we have efficiently strengthened even the most deconditioned patients because we are able to educate them about how to make better treatment choices, choices that take into account both their own goals and those that create realistic expectations. I don't get cornered as easily into performing surgery for cases that do not have a high success rate (like Dave, my 30-year-old patient we discussed in the Introduction). The bonus is that over time I have found that strengthening helps multiple conditions that I had previously thought could be addressed only surgically.

Strengthening helps multiple conditions.

To succeed, I have learned that you need practitioners with complementary skills—an integrated platform of specialized trainers, exercise physiologists, and spine specialists—to work closely together for customized and integrated care to ensure the best patient outcomes. Unlike many existing methods that focus on relief of pain through passive treatments such as ultrasound, ice, massage, or active release treatments, the goal of the multi-disciplinary team at SpineZone is to improve long-term stability, posture, and strength for improved function. There is a protocol in place for trainers to help patients sequentially strengthen and mobilize their spines in a measurable way.

They also provide me and my other staff with individualized patient feedback if progress stalls so that we can adjust their rehabilitation, try a focused injection or medication, or explain what is occurring to increase their confidence about choosing non-operative treatment over surgery—just as I wish someone had done for me.

The thing is, surgery *can* sometimes provide dramatic results. Surgery is better for some conditions rather than others. For elective surgery, the only way to know what is right for you as an individual is to become informed about the options and fully engage in targeted strengthening to see where it takes you first.

When you choose a surgeon, be sure that he or she understands and fully appreciates all of you: your goals, your dreams, your aspirations. Make sure he or she asks about your current activity level: What can you do now, what can't you do, and what do you wish you could do? It is vitally important that your surgeon understands how a potential surgery could affect your individual needs and lifestyle.

For an elective surgery, put yourself in someone's hands who does more than look at an X-ray and explain a procedure—someone who will not rush a discussion with you about your alternatives, but instead will ensure you have realistic long-term expectations, whether you choose to undergo a procedure or forgo it. Perhaps most importantly, make sure that the surgeon you select is well versed in and connected with the best non-operative treatments available. There is a great adage that my favorite mentors repeated to me often: "Good surgeons know how to operate, better ones when to operate, and the best when *not* to operate." It takes not only experience, but humility, wisdom, and courage not to intervene.

Finally, as I mentioned in the Introduction, approach your discussions with your surgeon and your ultimate decision with an eye toward your long-term health and future quality of life *even if it costs you time and more money out of pocket.* Never agree to undergo a surgery that you don't feel good about just because "it's what insurance will pay for." Alternatively, don't waste your money on unproven treatments that don't empower you to take control of your condition. Your future well-being hinges on making the right decision *for you*—and there is no better investment in terms of your time or your finances.

CHAPTER 2

YOU ARE A UNIQUE INDIVIDUAL

"Today you are you! This is truer than true! There is no one alive who is you-er than you!"

—Dr. Seuss

An interesting thing about patients is that they don't always follow text-books in how they respond to various medical conditions. In western medicine, we categorize and classify conditions based on what we observe over time and our understanding of anatomy through dissections and surgery. But the truth is that everyone is actually slightly different, and these differences matter when it comes to understanding your condition and obtaining the best treatment.

We are not only different thanks to our genetic makeup, but also because of our unique environment. The information embedded in our genes, called our genotype, carries the range of possibilities for a certain trait. Take for example our eye color. We inherited a set of genes from each parent that form the palette from which our eye color is determined.

The expression of that gene information, called the phenotype, is the visible or observable expression of the genes. Even though our genes provide us the raw blue and yellow color in our eyes (the genotype), our body can use as much or little of those colors to create the actual color we express to the outside (our phenotype). Our eyes could look pure blue, yellow, or any combination of green depending on how much of each color is mixed in to create us. Similarly, in many traits such as height or weight, our environment and experiences significantly affect the final result, or expression of that gene.

Likewise, when it comes to certain diseases—such as disc disease—we may be genetically "coded" with a palette that includes increased susceptibility toward disc degeneration. However, based on the unique circumstances of our lives, we may use only a small portion of that palette and actually not develop significant disc degeneration. Considering this interplay between genotype and environment, we can conclude that our genes are only a *part* of who we are.

We all know that we should eat well and exercise. Some of us, knowing that heart disease runs in our family, may think it pointless to eat well and get active if we are just going to get sick anyway. So why should we choose to take better care of ourselves? Quite simply, because if we do so, we can selectively employ the genes that keep our hearts healthy.

Multiple studies have confirmed the association between genetic influences and spinal disorders such as disc degeneration and scoliosis, a curvature of the spine.[1,2] While we think of genetics as predictive, it's not definitive. We know that the daughter of a woman who has scoliosis is at increased risk of having the same condition, as is the son of a man who has struggled with stenosis and severe disc disease. Yet, these individuals may not actually develop the disease of their parents. By being aware of our genetic tendencies, we can monitor individuals and take early action even before a disease manifests.

> *While we think of genetics as predictive, it's not definitive.*

Your Destiny Can Be Shaped

The exciting news is that our physical reality is largely determined by factors that are actually within our control. This means that our fates are not predetermined. Individuals with the same genes for body height, for example, may still vary greatly with respect to their height. In other words, some will be taller or shorter than others. You can't predict your phenotype from your genotype alone.

As I have stated before, environment matters greatly. Studies increasingly document the important role of the environment in whether or not an individual will get a disease. One spine study of identical twins showed that their disc degeneration was genetically determined only between 30 and 50 percent of the time, which still means at least half of a person's likelihood to actually develop disc degeneration is due to environmental factors.[3] This accounts for a huge window of opportunity to improve one's health.

Degenerative disc disease is, in fact, already recognized to be a complex disease determined by the interplay between genes and an accumulation of environmental factors.[4] These external factors can include a vast array of strains and trauma, postural factors, occupational exposure, medications, diet, sports activities, spinal injuries, cigarette smoking, and atherosclerosis (the build-up of fats on artery walls) that overlay normal changes associated with aging.[5]

Studies regarding scoliosis show that the daughter of a woman who has scoliosis will develop scoliosis less than one-third of the time, even though she inherited her mother's scoliosis gene.[6,7] Her brother will have a lower probability of only 1 in 10 of developing scoliosis.

This conclusion is remarkable. Even though we have the gene for a condition, it may not turn on, and whether it turns on or not is often determined by environmental conditions.

Here is the bottom line: To a very large degree, our destiny is in our own hands through the choices we make. Just as that person who is genetically prone to heart attacks can reduce his chance of experiencing one by following a healthy diet, so too can we reduce the chance of developing a spine disorder by stacking the environmental factors in our favor.

To a very large degree, our destiny is in our own hands through the choices we make.

A person with inflammatory arthritis, for instance, may modify his diet, perform activities that keep the inflammation at bay, and choose an occupation that doesn't involve heavy labor. Another person who is prone to disc disease can prevent its development and progression by not succumbing to a sedentary job, maintaining ideal body weight, and strengthening the muscles that support the disc.

My own parents both have spondylolisthesis, a condition in which a vertebra in the spine slips out of the proper position to create structural instability. My mother, who still practices part-time as a physician, experiences back and leg pain and will likely need surgery at some point. Fortunately, this is a condition for which surgery is very well suited.

And yet my father, who has spent most of his life gardening and has farmed almonds in the Central Valley of California, has virtually no pain. Just like those Midwestern farmers I studied early in my career who seem to defy their spinal defects through a lifetime of physical activity, my dad still plays tennis, bends, digs, and lifts things that even I find challenging to lift, all without pain!

Sitting Is the New Smoking

Now that we know just how important environment truly is in the expression of your genes, let's discuss a few factors that can majorly affect your spine health and, in turn, your back and neck pain.

Sitting is the new smoking.

I have had many patients who suffer from chronic back pain tell me that they feel they are destined to have surgery since their parents also had severe degenerative discs and suffered from back pain their whole adult lives.

I can't emphasize enough the importance of not getting stuck in this frame of mind. As we already discussed in this chapter, even though your genes may make you more predisposed to developing disc disease, you would be surprised by how much influence your activity level has on this process.

Perhaps one of the most surprising new findings on environmental factors is the negative impact that sitting has on spinal health. While we might assume that individuals with physically strenuous jobs are at increased risk, this is not necessarily so. One real culprit for back pain in many individuals is working long hours at a sedentary desk job. So, in a counterintuitive twist, office employees typing away at their desks—not laborers who lift and strain daily—can actually be more at risk with their necks and backs!

Dr. James Levine, director of the Mayo Clinic/Arizona State University Obesity Solutions Initiative, says, "Sitting is more dangerous than smoking, kills more people than HIV, and is more treacherous than parachuting. We are sitting ourselves to death."[8] (Yes, he is the researcher credited with coining the mantra "Sitting is the new smoking.")

In addition to increasing our risk for developing conditions like cancer, heart disease, and type 2 diabetes, sitting can be very bad for your back. The disc is the largest "avascular" structure in your body, meaning that most of it has no direct blood supply. Instead, nutrients seep into the spine, and waste products pump out of it. However, when you sit, you put constant pressure on the front part of the disc, which restricts the spine's ability to obtain those nutrients and pump out those waste products. So the longer you sit, the more you create a noxious environment in your spine, which leads to disc degeneration.

The other problem with sitting is that over time, bad posture puts unequal strain on your discs, exposing them to injury. Imagine that each disc is an evenly spread but particularly packed peanut butter and jelly sandwich. When you sit, your lower back loses its normal protective curve, called "lordosis," and the back assumes more of a "C" curve. The more you sit, the more unequal strain is placed on the back portion of the disc, which can tear, causing disc herniations. This is similar to you trying to take a bite out of the sandwich, and as a result, squeezing the peanut butter and jelly out of the back of the sandwich.

In this sandwich analogy, you would end up with a messy floor, but when it comes to your spine, the disc is right next to your nerves, so when it tears, its contents squeeze out, causing back pain, spasm, and sciatica.

Remember, the back is made of multiple joints. And just like any overworked joint that suffers from too many repetitive movements without recovery—a knee pounding on moguls on a ski slope, for example—you will eventually feel the effects of the excess wear and tear caused by sitting.

The fact is, humans did not evolve to sit for long periods in front of computers. As hunter/gatherers, when we sat, we sat on the ground in a cross-legged position that allowed for nice rotation of the hips and flexion in our knees. This improved range of motion not only nourished those joints, but also decreased the pressure on the spine. And we didn't sit for long; we alternated sitting with running, climbing, walking, and crawling movements.

> *Humans did not evolve to sit for long periods in front of computers.*

What's worse, your mind is engaged with work or other distractions when you sit at a computer. Because of this, you are far less likely to notice that you are sitting for a very long time in a position that puts strain on your back. In some cultures, people still spend more time squatting or sitting on the ground, and as a result, they have far fewer problems with joint flexibility.

Tips for Sitting Properly

If your job requires you to spend hours sitting at a desk, don't despair! While spending years sitting at a desk for 40 hours a week is in no way ideal, you can still prevent the bad posture that leads to chronic back or neck pain.

First of all, it's important to sit *correctly*. As I will describe in this section, I have learned some simple sitting modifications that have helped my patients and me.[9]

It is imperative to understand how to maintain correct posture for protection of your neck, torso, and low back. You may be tempted to buy an "ergonomic" chair that promises to fix your posture and relieve back pain. Know right away that many expensive chairs are made in such a way that the pelvis gets tucked at an angle that forces the spine to rest in an unhealthy "C" shaped posture when viewed from the side. While you may be able to find a chair that doesn't allow this to happen, know that there are less expensive ways to prevent this damaging "C" posture.

Based on the anatomy of the disc and muscles, there are ways to prevent prolonged episodes of sitting from resulting in pain. Your goal is to supply good nutrition to the discs and to maintain the spine in a position that doesn't strain the muscles or other soft tissues of the spine.

To attain this goal, it is important to understand and control the position of your pelvis while you sit at your desk (or anywhere, really). This is where proper alignment begins—at the pelvis. Prolonged sitting often results in the pelvis rotating backward (this is called retroversion), which causes the spine and the entire back to fall into the familiar "C" shaped posture. (See the left image on the following page to view a retroverted pelvis and the resulting poor posture.)

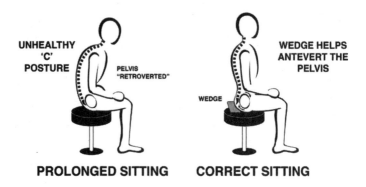

PROLONGED SITTING   CORRECT SITTING

You can combat the tendency to "slump" by rotating your pelvis out of retroversion. When the pelvis is maintained in a more anteverted position (see the right image in the diagram), it automatically neutralizes the lower back and keeps it away from the unhealthy "C" posture.

There are a few ways to correct this problem. You can either roll up a small towel or place a small pillow behind the buttocks to help rotate the pelvis forward. Or, if you prefer, you can purchase a wedge pillow designed for this purpose.

Aside from using a wedge, you can use the flesh and muscle from the buttocks to help rotate the pelvis to its proper position. To do this, lean forward and to the left. Then grab the flesh of the right buttocks and pull it up and back. Do the same to the other side. You will feel your muscles gently propelling you forward and providing support.

Next, work your way up the spine to address the remaining issues that contribute to back pain. Start by rolling one shoulder slightly forward, then lifting it up to the ear. Then roll the shoulder back and down as far as you comfortably can. It is as if you are trying to place your shoulder blade in your back pocket. Notice the ease you find in this position. Now, do the same with your other shoulder.

Finally, let's lengthen and properly position the head and neck. One way to do this is to imagine having an object on the top of your head. Now push up against this imaginary object while keeping it balanced. This exercise automatically levels your head and lengthens your neck muscles. Alternatively, you can tuck your chin back while keeping your head level. Or you can even grasp the base of your skull and gently pull your head up to lengthen the neck muscles. The goal here is to be able to line up your ear with your shoulder and pelvis.

Performing the sequence above allows you to maintain good posture without having to try to forcefully hold the posture with your muscles. You shouldn't at any point feel like you are gripping your muscles into an awkward formation. Above all, try to find a place of gentle comfort as you take these steps to align your spine. Repeat this process any time you notice that your posture is incorrect or whenever you feel pain, and reset your position periodically as you notice it slipping.

Further Modifications

There are additional modifications you can make while driving or sitting in chairs that helps to unburden the spinal discs and facilitate better back health. This is called "stretch sitting."[10] While sitting, bend forward slightly to lengthen the back of your spine. With both hands, push up on some part of the chair, arm rest, or cushion so that you can further lengthen your spine.

Finally, "lock" this lengthened posture onto the back of the chair. Additionally, you can lengthen your neck against the headrest to provide gentle traction. See the images below.

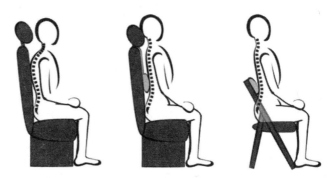

Image A: Standard sitting in a car. Image B: Securing a cushion in the appropriate spot (needs to have straps so it doesn't drop) and lowering the headrest to lie under the base of the skull allows a "stretch" of both the lumbar and cervical spine, respectively. Note that the cushion and headrest are placed at the top of the curves of your lower back and neck and are meant to provide a surface against which there is friction to provide the stretch. Image C: You can simulate this "stretch" sitting in any seat by locking the lengthened posture onto the back of the chair. For your neck, imagine that you are pushing your head to the sky (while keeping your head level). This will lengthen your neck safely as long as you don't tilt your head. For more information and free workshops, visit www.gokhalemethod.com.

Taking Frequent Breaks

Let's take a moment here to talk about sharks. (Yes, *sharks*!) You may be aware that sharks exist in a constant state of motion, which continually forces oxygen-rich water into their systems. If a shark were to stop moving, it wouldn't be able to breathe and would immediately suffocate. It is important to think of your spinal discs in the same light. Like sharks, which must swim in order to survive, your discs require daily movement in order to stay healthy and viable.

When you must sit for long intervals, it is very important to take frequent breaks. This practice either assures that your posture hasn't slipped or totally resets your posture when you get up, stretch, and walk around a bit.

I recommend that you take breaks from sitting every 30 minutes. At the very least be sure to stand up and move around every hour. Go for a short walk (even if it is just down the hall!) and consider doing some light stretching, just to ensure that your blood is flowing. And when you do sit down again to work, take a moment to observe your posture and use the exercises described above to make subtle adjustments. They will garner big results.

The Role of Inflammation

Another major factor that contributes to back and neck pain is the presence of inflammation in the joints and tissues of the spine. One marker of inflammation in the body is the presence of pain. One effective way to combat joint problems in general, and specifically chronic back and neck pain, is ridding the body of extra inflammation.

In order to understand the role inflammation plays in pain, let's first take a look at arthritis. What does a diagnosis of arthritis mean anyway? The inflammation of a joint—no more and no less.

Individual factors, such as underlying inflammatory processes, create pain and stiffness in arthritis patients. There are many diseases and hypersensitivities in which your body's immune system attacks its own tissues and organs, creating inflammation and joint destruction. These inflammatory arthritis conditions include rheumatoid arthritis and a disorder called ankylosing spondylitis that can cause vertebrae in the spine to fuse together. They generally result from a combination of genetic and environmental factors, many of which are unknown.

Even though having a close relative with rheumatoid arthritis likely increases a person's risk for developing the condition, there are multiple factors that remain in your control—and this point can't be emphasized enough.

Long-term smoking, for example, is a well-established risk factor for developing rheumatoid arthritis.[11] In fact, smoking is also associated with more severe signs and symptoms in people who have the disease. The habit is also a big risk factor in developing back pain even in people without inflammatory arthritis. Smoking cessation is the most easily identifiable, preventable factor, but there are likely other triggers, such as occupational exposure to certain kinds of dust or fibers, and viral or bacterial infections.

Another factor that is completely in your control is your diet. Even though there are no specific, globally accepted dietary guidelines for people suffering from rheumatoid arthritis, there are certain guidelines I find very beneficial for patients who are in pain. The goal is to eat a diet that reduces inflammation.

For example, eating a diet rich in omega-3 fatty acids, known antioxidants, and phytochemicals can show improvements in pain, morning stiffness, disease activity, physical function, and improved vitality in patients with rheumatoid arthritis.[12] A key compound found in extra-virgin olive oil, oleocanthal, has a significant impact on inflammation and helps reduce cartilage damage. Oleocanthal has been shown to prevent the production of pre-inflammatory COX-1 and COX-2 enzymes, similar to how ibuprofen works.[13] In fact, about 3 ½ Tbsp. of virgin olive oil is equal to a 200-mg tablet of ibuprofen in terms of its anti-inflammatory effect. Be aware, though, that this amount of oil has more than 400 calories, so it's a good idea to use in moderation to avoid gaining weight.

There are other dietary habits that could significantly help shape the expression of your inflammatory arthritis. Although they are not for everybody, vegetarian or vegan diets can significantly impact inflammation in general and rheumatoid arthritis in particular.[14] Researchers have also found that an antioxidant in green tea significantly reduces the severity of arthritis.[15] Finally, high-fiber diets, including foods such as oatmeal, brown and wild rice, beans, barley, and quinoa, can help reduce C-reactive protein levels (a marker of inflammation).[16] (There are also studies showing the benefit of whole-food, plant-based diets in alleviating symptoms of osteoarthritis.)[17]

Why am I focusing on rheumatoid arthritis in a book aimed at helping alleviate back pain in readers who may not suffer from that disease? I want to illustrate to you how dietary choices can affect even a very strong inflammatory disease. The foods that we choose to eat contribute to our overall health, for better or for worse. I encourage you to think carefully about your diet and whether you could be eating healthier foods than you currently do.

The Arthritis Foundation recommends a diet that aims to reduce and control inflammation in the body that closely resembles the guidelines of the popular Mediterranean diet. I agree with their recommendations, which is why I have summarized the guidelines I've found most helpful in helping patients control their own inflammation and thus their pain.

FIGHTING INFLAMMATION WITH FOOD: 10 GUIDELINES TO TRY RIGHT NOW

1. **Avoid processed foods.** Yes, they're convenient and tasty, but processed foods are full of unhealthy fats and artificial ingredients. Though it is difficult, try to avoid chips, cookies, and packaged snacks. Reach for whole, fresh foods instead. And if you can, choose frozen vegetables over canned.

2. **Get your fiber fix.** Dietary fiber can be found in a wealth of vegetable sources. It lowers your levels of C-reactive protein, a marker of inflammation found in your blood. Choose carrots, broccoli, artichokes, spinach, and other high-fiber veggies daily.

3. **Focus on fish.** Fish is a very healthy form of protein. Eat salmon, tuna, sardines, and cold

water fish. These types of fish contain omega-3 fatty acids, which reduce inflammation.

4. **Drizzle on the olive oil.** Aim for up to three tablespoons a day of extra-virgin olive oil. EVOO is a great source of monosaturated fat, antioxidants, and oleocanthal, which is a compound that lowers pain and inflammation.

5. **Get plenty of fruits and vegetables.** Colorful fruits and vegetables are full of antioxidants that support your immune system. Eat plenty of blueberries, blackberries, cherries, strawberries, spinach, kale, and broccoli. Try to get a serving of vegetables at every meal, and remember that fruit makes a tasty "dessert."

6. **Bring on the beans.** Beans are good for your health and your budget. This affordable staple food is full of fiber, protein, folic acid, and minerals. They contain antioxidants and anti-inflammatory compounds.

7. **Eat walnuts, pine nuts, pistachios, or almonds.** Nuts provide a healthy serving of monosaturated fat, protein, and fiber, too. They will keep you full between meals and help fight inflammation.

8. **Eat onions.** They are full of antioxidants and may also reduce inflammation, heart disease risk, and LDL cholesterol levels (the "bad" type). Add them to your dishes whenever you can.

9. **Enjoy a glass of wine.** Red wine contains resveratrol, a compound that may reduce inflammation. While it is probably okay to drink moderate amounts of alcohol, be sure to check with your physician to determine how much you can safely drink, if any.

10. **Consider reducing nightshades.** Some experts believe that nightshade vegetables—tomatoes, potatoes, peppers, eggplant—may increase inflammatory responses in the body. However, the research is not conclusive. Try eliminating nightshades from your diet for a month and see if your pain levels improve.

More information on the tenets I've listed in the above sidebar, as well as other tips and guidelines, can be found on the Arthritis Foundation's website at www.arthritis.org.

The Mystery and Magic of Neural Pathways

Yet another factor in determining our individual reality is how our unique neural pathways are wired. We know through the example of cognitive-behavioral therapy—which we will examine more in the next chapter—that new thoughts can create new behaviors. When we practice pairing new stimuli—such as a pleasant image instead of an unpleasant image while we think about a difficult relative—we can effectively change our relationship with this individual.

When we train ourselves to pair the image of that difficult mother-in-law with the smell of her tasty apple pie instead of her complaining tone, for example, we get a nice fresh feeling when we think of her, instead of a guttural "ugh!" That's because we have rewired our neural pathways; in this case, a new connection is made to the brain area that elicits all of the great emotion associated with the smell of our favorite dessert instead of the brain area that gets agitated and increases our heart rate.

This was not common knowledge even 10 years ago. But thanks to the rapidly advancing field of neuroscience, we now know that the human brain has the capacity to reshape and rewire itself in response to what it senses from its surroundings, not just in infancy, but throughout our adult lives, based on our experiences. Each time we have an experience, there is a distinct physical change in the way in which brain cells attach to other brain cells. Just as we constantly create new neural pathways in the brain, so too does this occur in the body through many different mechanisms.

Each time we have an experience,
there is a distinct physical change in
the way in which brain cells attach to
other brain cells.

The Psychophysiological Side of Pain

Many, many factors come together to determine an individual's unique experience and tolerance for pain as well as their ability to cope with it. These include:

Physiological makeup. The first thing to understand about pain is that we differ in our physiological makeups. Studies show that individuals who have more gray matter in their brains tend to be more sensitive to pain, for instance.[18] (Gray matter is made up of all of the brain cells and their interconnections, while white matter is like the "subway" of the brain, connecting regions of grey matter to one another.)

The brain also determines the emotion we attach to pain. That's because there are two different systems that process pain in the brain. One identifies where the pain is coming from, how intense it is, and the type of pain (i.e., aching, stabbing). The second system is the emotional side of pain—the part that makes us judge the pain as unbearable. While the brain can literally decide to turn down the volume on pain or turn it up, scientists are still working to understand this mechanism for regulation.

But again, you can control the grip that pain has on your life. You are not destined to suffer from pain more than others just because your brain is more sensitized to it.

In one study on pain, genetic factors could explain only 30 percent of how individuals perceived pain and only 20 percent for chemical burn pain.[19] Since only a small percentage of our perception of pain is determined by our genetics, the vast majority is due to other factors that are unique to each of us. And for those of us who experience more pain, we can still minimize it by promoting positive emotions over negative ones, to ensure we feel calm, safe, and supported.

Thoughts and expectations. Many simultaneous thoughts swirl through our heads and are often competing for our attention. Which processes are allowed to win this competition depends on how strong the sensation is and how much we focus on it. Tasks requiring subjects to direct their attention to something other than pain frequently produce reductions in pain. So, at any point in time, some of the variation in the intensity of the pain we perceive can be attributed to which thoughts a person generates and how focused he or she is on those thoughts.

The influence of our *expectations* on pain can also be profound. It has been shown that when people expect less pain, they perceive up to 50 percent less pain.[20] In fact, most people seem to have a high tolerance for what they might consider "productive pain"—when a woman chooses a natural childbirth, for instance. And yet, this same woman may experience tremendous pain with an ankle sprain or surgery.

> *The influence of our* expectations *on pain can be profound.*

Likewise, many men who are active sports enthusiasts don't register much pain when they charge into a 250-pound opponent on the football field because it was an elective decision to play. And yet, these same men are often highly anxious or agitated and report high levels of pain when exposed to a needle stick for a blood test or when an IV is inserted.

Thoughts and expectations are also the basis for the placebo effect. (Placebos, as you may know, are harmless pills, perceptions, circumstances, procedures, or medicines that are often used as controls in studies to compare against an intervention with a true therapeutic effect.) Placebos provide a clear demonstration of how our perceived senses can be altered by previously accepted thoughts. In fact, placebo analgesia (i.e., a sugar pill) can activate both the spinal cord and numerous brain regions similar to an actual pain medication.[21]

Indeed, the growing field of "epigenetics" studies all of these very factors that influence gene expression. It turns out that a whole host of things turn the genes we have inherited on and off. These include diet, exercise, and environmental toxins, as well as our thoughts, feelings, and beliefs. This only further supports just how much control you actually have in determining whether your back pain impacts the rest of your life—or becomes a thing of the past.

In his book, *The Genie in Your Genes,* researcher Dawson Church, PhD, writes, "Your body reads your mind. Science is discovering that while we may have a fixed set of genes in our chromosomes, which of those genes is active has a great deal to do with our subjective experiences, and how we process them."

In one study at Ohio State University, researchers found that blisters healed more slowly in the bodies of study participants who had engaged in argumentative conversations with their spouse versus those who had engaged in neutral conversations.[22] This is because the signal to your wound-healing genes (and hence, the repair process) slows down when the body's energy is being overrun by stress hormones.

The Ohio State study showed the sensitivity of wound healing to everyday stressors; in this case, an unpleasant marital discussion of only a half-hour slowed wound healing by an entire day. Imagine what happens when more frequent and amplified stressors accelerate the range of disorders that occur with aging, such as the hardening of our arteries or the stretching and sagging of our skin. Conversely, when the body is not preparing itself for a perceived threat, its energy is readily available for healing.

Gender and hormones. There are other biological mechanisms at work with pain tolerance as well. Studies show that our perceptions of pain can differ based on our gender and specific hormones. We know that women's bodies produce a hormone called oxytocin that improves pain tolerance and aids in forgetting pain post-childbirth. Oxytocin is famously called the "love hormone," a brain peptide known to promote positive inter-social relations. It makes people like one another, especially in intimate relationships.

> *Our perceptions of pain can differ based on our gender and specific hormones.*

New mothers are awash in oxytocin (which is involved in the labor process), and it is believed that the hormone promotes bonding between mother and infant. We can also modulate the effects of oxytocin. In fact, oxytocin, when delivered via the nose, has been studied as a treatment for headaches.[23] Exercise also increases the levels of this remarkable hormone.[24]

Cortisol. Pain perception can also depend on our individual levels of cortisol, a life-sustaining hormone produced by our bodies that regulates our blood sugar, levels of inflammation, and sleep, to name just a few of the vital functions it performs.

Cortisol varies in a fascinating daily rhythm that is highest in the morning (in healthy individuals) to promote wakefulness and lowest in the evening. This is also why many individuals experience more pain at night when cortisol levels are at their lowest. The amount of cortisol and its rhythm vary highly from individual to individual.

The good news is: You can change your level of cortisol with exercise.[25] When you exercise, you naturally increase your levels of cortisol and naturally experience less pain overall.

Physical fitness. When it comes to exercise, studies show that people who are more physically fit tend to tolerate pain better. In one 2014 study, a team of Australian researchers measured pain threshold and pain tolerance in a group of non-athletes, and then turned half of them into athletes and remeasured their pain threshold and pain tolerance after six weeks of training.[26] The result? People who trained increased their pain tolerance by a whopping 20 percent, while their pain threshold didn't change. In other words, these individuals found a given sensation just as painful as they previously did, but after their level of fitness increased, they could handle that level of discomfort for significantly longer.

When you exercise, your body releases chemicals called endorphins.[27] The chemicals are responsible for the euphoria of the "runner's high." This high is similar to that produced by morphine or other opioid medications. In fact, our body's own endorphins bind to the same nerve receptors that bind opioid pain medications. Unlike the medications, though, our body's endorphins do *not* lead to addiction or dependence. (However, they may lead you to exercise more often to experience the pleasant effect!) The added benefit of these medications is that they are also sedatives that reduce stress and ward off anxiety and feelings of depression.

I find these physiological factors in the perception of pain to be remarkable. Not only can we turn on or off the genes that promote healing through our thoughts, but we can also rewire our perception of pain. Equally importantly, we can directly influence the levels of hormones like oxytocin, cortisol, and endorphins with exercise, which in turn decreases our perception of pain. Exercise is beneficial in so many, many ways, which we will examine more closely in upcoming chapters.

We can rewire our perception of pain.

There is no truly objective way to measure pain. So when we consider the many reasons we experience pain and all the ways it can be experienced differently among individuals, it should give us pause as we consider surgery or succumb to the feeling that pain is out of our control.

While the unpleasant sensation you feel is surely legitimate, an intervention to treat it must first consider the underlying pathology, your function, and your current physical and emotional state. (In other words, how fit are you? How much has your condition progressed?

What are your expectations? And how well are you coping?)

You have more power than you think to change your perception of pain. For this reason, it is important not to make a hasty decision—because surgery may not cure your symptoms.

Response to narcotics. Despite the fact that, as established above, it's quite possible to increase the body's own levels of natural painkillers, many patients request, and many physicians still prescribe, opioids to help individuals with chronic pain. Our high-pressure sedentary lifestyles make us increasingly prone to chronic back and neck pain. And once that pain kicks in, exercise is curtailed even further and the body stops producing its natural opioids. We really crave these opioids, and if the body isn't producing them, it's understandable that patients seek out a pharmaceutical alternative. Be careful to avoid this trap!

If your situation warrants the use of long-term narcotics, it is vital that you proceed with caution. In addition to the mind-numbing effect and tolerance issues, which we will discuss in Chapter 3, it is important to know that individual receptiveness to opioids differs greatly. Some quickly become addicted; some develop significant side effects such as dizziness, nausea, or constipation; and even others' bodies metabolize and breakdown the opioids so quickly that high doses are required. After all, you are a unique being. All the factors that make you *you* influence your reaction to variables like opioids.

How can you know if you are one of those people who could experience severe complications with the use of such pain medications? Up until very recently, there was no way to know. Every patient is typically prescribed a standard starting dose to see how they respond. But a few companies are now in the process of developing genetic testing where your DNA can be sequenced based on a saliva sample that can provide information about your sensitivities. As research progresses, hopefully more people can use tests like these to learn whether prescription pills are really worth the risks that they pose.

The Future of Personalized Medicine

One day, in the not too distant future, doctors will be able to customize your medical care by making treatment decisions based on what they specifically know about your unique DNA based on testing. In fact, personalized medicine is already here on a small scale.

Doctors will customize your care by
making decisions based on what they
know about your unique DNA.

To date, this has typically involved genetic testing to determine a patient's responsiveness to drugs, as mentioned above. In fact, we've learned that some patients are "ultra-rapid metabolizers." This means that the enzymes in their livers work much more quickly than those in other patients when they take a drug like codeine. (Codeine is relatively inactive until it is metabolized into its active form, morphine.) While 10 percent of that dose typically becomes available to the body of a person with an average metabolism, fully 40 percent becomes quickly available to the body of an ultra-rapid metabolizer.

This "rush" of narcotic can usually be tolerated by younger patients, but will give a rapid high and may predispose them to abuse. Such a rapid infusion of morphine is even more acutely dangerous in older patients as it can lead to respiratory depression. So the opportunity to determine a person's metabolism before prescribing a drug has important implications for safety.

Conversely, in some people the body breaks down drugs more quickly, rendering them less effective. This can make needed drugs ineffective in some patients. It also is the reason why some "tolerate" their alcohol better than others; their livers are more effective at removing the alcohol from the bloodstream.

Laboratory tests have also become much more sophisticated in their ability to determine a detailed list of possible cross-reactions between medications. This is also welcome news. The truth is that when a person takes six medications, the chance of a significant cross-reaction is increased up to 95 percent.

Soon such labs will also be able to determine the probability that a patient will become dependent on or addicted to a medication. Thanks to these types of advances in biotechnology, physicians will soon have abundantly more information to be selective about their prescribing for the benefit of their patients. However, because we are still very early in using personalized genetic information to help us prescribe narcotic pain medication appropriately, we must be cautious in allowing the chronic usage of such a dangerous class of medication.

We are still in the infancy of the revolution toward personalized medicine. Until that day comes when we can reliably test for the many factors at work in an individual's pain for a scientific approach to treatment, we must make conscious lifestyle choices to treat our bodies well, given our genetic predispositions. Just as we can get an extra 50,000 miles out of an older car if we perform regular maintenance, so too can we enjoy pain-free good health into our twilight years when it comes to our spine.

Remodeling Your Back

Are we destined to rapidly lose function or experience increasing pain as we age? I believe the answer is no—*if* we take steps to prevent this from happening. Specifically, strengthening is critical if we wish to enjoy good health into our twilight years.

First, understand that we are destined to lose some muscle mass as we age. Beginning at age 30, most people lose about 1 percent muscle mass every year, and this loss of strength can increase exponentially with age. The Arthritis Foundation notes that we are likely to lose between 20 and 40 percent of our muscle and 30 percent of our strength from age 50 to 70.[28] This even happens to the strongest of us, as indicated by the world weightlifting records for men being 30 percent lower in the 60-year-old age bracket as compared to the 30-year-old bracket. The problem is that with inactivity, this muscle wasting can accelerate to 3-5 percent per year, which eventually leads to dysfunction.

We are likely to lose between 20 and 40 percent of our muscle and 30 percent of our strength from age 50 to 70.

Sarcopenia is an accelerated form of muscle wasting. It has been defined as the loss of skeletal muscle mass and strength that accelerates with advancing age. Recent estimates indicate that approximately 45 percent of the older U.S. population is affected by sarcopenia.[29] The risk of disability—such as challenges with mobility, risk of falls, and decreased daily functions like walking, climbing stairs, and getting out of chairs—is 1.5-4.6 times higher in older patients with sarcopenia than those with normal muscle mass.[30] As a result, approximately 20 percent of the elderly U.S. population is functionally disabled.[31] That equates to 18 million people in 2010.

The news isn't all that bad though. While we can't completely stop this aging process, we can (and should) do a lot to slow it down. The key to slowing this decline is resistance training (as well as a dietary component, which we'll discuss momentarily). Landmark research many years ago showed that previously sedentary postmenopausal women who lifted weights twice a week for a year could increase their muscle strength by about 80 percent.[32] The exercises traded fat for muscle, improved their balance, and built strength and small but significant amounts of bone density.

We will further address resistance training in later chapters, but for now be aware that the muscle-boosting effects of proper exercise may be limited without an adequate dietary intake of protein, according to a recent study.[33] We need to ingest about 25 to 30 grams of protein per meal, the amount in four ounces of lean meat or a three-egg and cheese omelet to maximally stimulate muscle buildup when and if we work out. But don't overdo it, since eating 12 ounces of beef did not provide any extra benefits to the study participants and only added more calories. Nor should you try to consume only 10 to 20 grams of protein at breakfast and lunch, then have 60 grams at dinner, since this will result in less muscle protein buildup than getting 30 grams at each meal.

Supplements of leucine, an amino acid, have also been shown to be promising to maximally stimulate muscle protein synthesis.[34] And timing is important. Research has shown that this amount of protein, when eaten immediately after a resistance-training workout, boosted the body's muscle-building rate by 50 percent in both young and older people.[35]

Not only can we decrease the natural loss of muscle mass and bone density, we can also reshape our joints. A terrific yet extreme example of this remodeling capacity is Floyd Landis, a world-class cyclist who finished ninth in the 2005 Tour de France race and finished first in the 2006 race before being stripped of his title when he was eventually found guilty of doping. He suffered from a very painful hip ailment, osteonecrosis, which had resulted from a fracture in a 2002 cycling accident.

Osteonecrosis occurs when a portion of the hip ball loses its blood supply and collapses. This results in a very irregular ball joint that doesn't fit into the socket. The amazing thing about Landis is that through his training, he was able to remodel a groove in his joint that only "ached" when he pedaled. He couldn't walk even short distances without severe pain, but won the most grueling road test in the world.

There is no reason to think that the spine is any different from the hip or knee in the way it can respond to appropriate exercise. The important point to understand here is that your body is more resilient than you think, and even though you may be dealt a few less than desirable genes, how you treat your body has a big impact on your function and enjoyment of life. By actively using the innate intelligence of your body—the many mechanisms it already has in place to remodel, stay strong, and combat pain—you can use these stimuli to your benefit instead of your detriment.

When we do specific exercises to strengthen the spine, we not only reduce the pain, but we prevent the progression of any problems by stabilizing the joint and increasing the nutritional blood supply to the disc. Remember, you have the power to determine your future, as we have seen. Your back and other joints are not static; they are indeed "moldable."

In fact, we can learn quite a bit from patients whose MRI or X-ray shows a severe structural deficit but experience no pain or functional problems. These individuals confirm for us that such anatomic abnormalities do not necessarily express themselves in a debilitating way and can in fact allow for a full and physically active life as long as we create the appropriate conditions for healing and avoid activities that could worsen the condition.

Before beginning a spinal rehabilitation program, it's important that the persons involved in your integrated training program understand the many unique factors about you that we have discussed in this chapter.

For example, if I see a patient with tightness of their cervical spinal canal so severe that it is causing progressive imbalance when walking, they will need modification of their rehabilitation program, close monitoring to detect even slight worsening, and appropriate referral for surgery. In such cases, standard personal training or physical therapy would be ill-advised as an alternative or to stave off surgery. If pushed to perform exercises that don't take into consideration the underlying condition, such patients could experience a long-term neurological deficit. And yet, it will still be important for them to work on improving their balance to regain function.

Slow Is Good

Until genetic testing catches up—and can predict whether we will develop things like tightness of the spinal canal (stenosis) or a disc problem and can help direct an early intervention or targeted medications that can eliminate pain—we must act with awareness of what we know about our bodies to keep them in good health.

We must act with awareness of what we know about our bodies.

In a recent NPR article titled "If slow is good for food, why not medicine?" the author questions the increasing rush to administer medical intervention and advocates more low-tech, high-touch medical care—and with good reason.[36] Just as the overuse of antibiotics is causing an epidemic of resistant bacteria and the overuse of medication in the elderly can cause bedsores, falls, and other hospital-acquired conditions, so too does our rush to intervene in chronic pain situations frequently cause harm to patients.

Patients with chronic degenerative spinal conditions do not face quick and impending doom if they don't have immediate surgery. And, in fact, much like the analogy of the tortoise and the hare, they frequently do better long-term with a slow, steady approach to improving strength and spinal health.

A San Francisco physician and slow medicine advocate, Dr. Victoria Sweet, notes that it's sometimes better to treat a sick patient the way a gardener treats an ailing plant, rather than the way a mechanic fixes a broken machine. As we have seen, there are many unique factors that make you *you*. So in the process of healing from chronic conditions, take it slowly so you can allow your individual healing capacity to manifest.

I find this to be particularly true for people with chronic back pain. For just as an injured plant can gradually heal itself, we can likewise harness the innate healing power of our bodies through a thoughtful, focused, and customized approach to regaining strength and function.

Key Learning Points: You Are a Unique Individual

1. We are unique because of the unique genes we inherited.
2. We are unique due to our individual life experiences.

3. We have the ability to shape our physical destiny with factors in our control, regardless of what our genes say.

4. We can reshape and rewire our brains by providing the correct stimuli.

5. We are harming ourselves by sitting too often. We need to find ways to be more active throughout the workday.

6. Inflammation plays a major role in pain. We can reduce our inflammation levels by eating a healthier diet.

7. To get the best medical treatment and to avoid common pitfalls, it is important for all those treating us to understand our medical states (e.g., inflammatory conditions, underlying diseases, differences in our thoughts).

8. There are many factors within our control that can affect our perception of pain.

9. By recognizing our physiological differences and sensitivities with respect to medications like narcotics, we can better assess risks appropriately and use caution when choosing to use them.

10. The field of spine health is changing quickly, so it is best to take it slow and not pursue an irreversible course too early.

CHAPTER 3

SUFFERING LIES WITHIN

> **"If you think you can do a thing or think you can't do a thing, you're right."**
>
> —Henry Ford

In 2009, on one of those rare but incredibly rainy days we sometimes have in San Diego, I was driving to work when my car hit a puddle on the freeway and immediately spun out. In the midst of the pouring rain, my car veered across all four freeway lanes and hit the guardrail. After the air bags deployed, I looked around to find myself in my car pointed in the wrong direction in the middle of the freeway and facing oncoming traffic. I was a bit dazed, but remarkably unhurt.

I sat there for a few moments until I got my wits about me. I remember taking pictures of the mangled car, feeling grateful that it did such a good job of protecting me. I took inventory of my body and had no trouble moving any of my limbs. My neck seemed to be fine.

The airbag had burned my arm a bit, but that was a minor inconvenience. So I called my wife to come get me. And since I felt fine, we went home.

But a couple of hours later, my thoughts began to race. I didn't actually remember anything between hitting the guardrail and spinning into the middle of the freeway, where I woke up facing opposing traffic that was slowing to gradually make its way around me. I wondered, *How long was I sitting there? Why couldn't I account for that time?*

My next thought was about Natasha Richardson, the actress and wife of Liam Neeson, who had sustained a head injury skiing in Quebec just a few months before. When paramedics and an ambulance arrived on the scene, Richardson said she felt fine and told them they weren't needed...so they left. But then, about three hours later in her hotel room, she began to complain of a headache. She was eventually transferred seven hours after her fall to the hospital in critical condition where she died of an "epidural hematoma" (an expanding blood clot in the brain) due to blunt impact to her head.

In medical school, they would have attributed Richardson's initial lack of symptoms to a "lucid interval." It's a lucid period of time where patients who have a head injury can talk and walk and basically feel fine—but then they rapidly deteriorate as the hematoma grows.

About the time that Natasha Richardson's accident came to mind, I noticed that the left side of my body seemed to be going numb and that the sensation seemed to be expanding. *Did I hit my head like she did?* I wondered. My one-sided body sensations seemed to be consistent with the type of injury she experienced. And so, as my low-level panic started to escalate, I felt it prudent to head straight to the emergency room. Guess what? As soon as I physically arrived in the ER—even before a doctor saw me—the numbness sensation completely left me. Coincidentally, my anxiety also went away.

In reality, of course, the abatement of my numbness and my anxiety were no coincidence. Once I stepped foot into the ER, I knew I was in a safe place. No matter what was wrong, I knew I could be helped immediately.

Needless to say, I did not have a blood clot in my head. But I was shocked by how quickly my thoughts and anxiety could manifest as physical symptoms in my body. This is something I see every day in patients I meet. Our thoughts *can* be relentless. And if we allow these types of repetitive thoughts to run unchecked when we are feeling worried, we can actually make ourselves physically ill.

This chapter is all about pain and the various ways that the mind can alter perceptions of it, for better or worse. Many people view pain as a one-sided nuisance that is almost always a causal reaction to an injury. Yet this is a huge simplification. While pain is often a symptom indicating that something is "wrong" in the body, there are many misconceptions regarding the nature of pain and how it should be treated. As we cover the different types of pain, you will learn to view pain itself in a different light.

Amy's Case: What Can Happen When the Mind Runs Wild

Many years ago, I examined Amy, a 22-year-old patient complaining of extreme weakness in one leg after she was involved in a rollover auto accident. Her fiancé, who had been driving, had been admitted to a different hospital with major internal injuries to his spleen, ribs, and lungs, among other organs. He had undergone emergency surgery and was still in the intensive care unit.

Despite taking X-rays, a CT scan, and MRI scan, the trauma surgeon could not identify a source for Amy's weakness. When I examined her, I found her to be very kind and amiable, but also jittery and quickly brought to tears. She was very distraught about her weakness and sure that she wouldn't walk again. And, in fact, she could not voluntarily flex her left knee or move her ankle. Since her MRI and CT scan showed no abnormalities and there were inconsistencies in her examination, I tried to distract her to determine if she was truly weak or if she could be suffering from some type of "conversion" disorder.

Conversion disorder is a condition that really highlights the mind-body connection. Patients with it suffer from neurological symptoms, such as numbness, blindness, or paralysis without a definable physical cause. It is thought that these symptoms arise in response to stressful situations that affect a patient's mental health.

In other words, the emotional charge of a painful experience is repressed as a way of managing the pain, but this emotional charge is somehow "converted" into neurological symptoms.

People who experience this phenomenon are not making up their symptoms. Even though these are sometimes dismissed as "in their head," the condition is real. It causes distress and cannot be turned on and off at will. The physical symptoms are thought to be an attempt to resolve the conflict the person feels inside.

Certain studies—those involving a special functional MRI (fMRI), which can actually show where activity is occurring in the brain—actually suggest a link between the emotional response of a patient with physical findings like Amy's, where there is unexplained right-sided paralysis. In a case report from 2007, a study was done to try to identify the cause of a young woman's right-sided weakness.[1] The patient was asked to recall traumatic events of the past, during which fMRI scanning was performed. The fMRI showed decreased activity in the area of the brain responsible for moving the right side of her body. This showed a correlation between her thoughts about a trauma and the "shutting off" of the area of the brain that moves a part of her body.

In Amy's case, because I did not find any evidence of a physical medical condition causing weakness, I reassured her that she would improve. Despite her request for additional studies, I recommended none to her trauma surgeon and she was discharged.

Two weeks later, Amy was admitted to the hospital again after tripping due to her weak leg, sustaining a head injury. This was her third admission, and each time she had complained of severe leg weakness. Noticing the same inconsistencies in her examination, I requested a psychiatric consultation.

It turns out that Amy was deeply distraught over the accident...so distraught that she had no memory of the event itself and admitted to the circumstances of the accident only once she was hypnotized. Apparently, she had distracted her fiancé at the time of the accident and was feeling a deep sense of guilt and regret over his injuries.

Soon after her fiancé had stabilized and was discharged from the hospital, I heard from the psychiatrist that her weakness had disappeared. While cases like these are extreme and rare, they are reported in the medical literature as a very real example of how our emotions can directly cause unintentional physical symptoms. In fact, studies indicate that 30 to 60 percent of patients in neurology clinics have unexplained physical symptoms.[2,3,4] How many of these patients could be having some sort of mind-body experience that we dismiss?

The Mind-Body Connection

We experience pain through a complex interplay between our minds and bodies. You have nerve cells in your spinal cord, for example, that transmit pain sensations that you feel in your body up into your brain stem. The impulse lands in a primary sensory area of the brain and then gets processed further in secondary areas. Even though a noxious emotional sensation starts in a different area of the brain, it is processed in much of the same secondary areas. Therefore the brain can be fooled into thinking that the body has sustained physical harm.

The brain also sends impulses down to the spinal cord that can inhibit the pain signal coming from the body. Why, you may wonder, does the body have built-in ways to actually decrease the pain sensation it feels? Think of how distracting and inhibiting it would be to feel every sensation as we are trying to concentrate on an important task or trying to run away from danger.

So as human beings, we are constantly experiencing a miraculous merge of sensations that are transmitted both *to* our bodies from our brains and *from* our bodies to our brains. It's an ebb and flow of thoughts and sensations that are really inseparable.

In addition to the many factors we have discussed that make you unique, your emotional life is one of the most powerful. Our thought processes that create anxiety, anger, and stress also manifest as sensations in the body. To take it a step further, I believe that our bodies "memorialize" these emotional reactions as physical sensations.

In other words, when you react to something—whether it's your disappointment when an expectation isn't met or a strong positive reaction to something you crave—I believe that the body experiences this disturbance in the form of physical sensations such as headaches or an upset stomach. And when we ignore the negative reactions, they may go deeply within us where they remain, ready to manifest again at the slightest cue.

For example, the first time I shared my different vision of where we would live with my wife or my differing vision of our practice with my partner, I reacted with mild discomfort to their conflicting opinions and the tension that resulted. I didn't accept things the way they were. Instead, I fought them and suppressed my discomfort. I thought that I could eventually change their views.

As a result, when one of those very same topics arose a few months later, and I realized that their views had not changed to my liking, I reacted much more passionately, with a deep area of discomfort in my neck and even felt a generalized sense of weakness. It is only by bringing awareness to what we are feeling—both emotionally and physically—that we can make the pain go away permanently.

John Sarno, a professor of rehabilitation medicine at New York University, first popularized the treatment of what he called "tension myositis syndrome," also known as mind-body medicine. He defines this as pain that results from deep, unresolved emotional issues that manifest as chronic back, neck, and limb pain, as well as gastrointestinal and dermatological issues—even repetitive strain injuries. He sees the pain as an unconscious distraction. Essentially, a person represses traumatic feelings through the help of this physical diversion.

To date, he's successfully treated more than 10,000 patients by "severing" this connection between the mind and physical pain. This is achieved not by use of a scalpel but through a process that involves learning to shift one's focus away from the physical symptom to the psychological issue using techniques like acceptance, goal setting, journaling, meditation, cultivating a positive attitude, and exercise. This process actually shuts down neural pathways that no longer serve us in favor of building new ones that do.

In one study of patients treated by Sarno, 88 percent of randomly selected patients stated they were free of pain one to three years after using these treatments. In another peer-reviewed study, results showed a 52 percent reduction in average pain intensity scores for 51 patients with chronic back pain.[5] Before the study, they had suffered with the pain for nine years.

Catastrophizing Pain (Everyone Does It!)

Similarly, psychologists and psychiatrists use the term "somatization disorder" to characterize significant complaints about bodily pain and other physical problems that cannot be fully explained by a medical condition upon examination. This disorder is commonly seen in patients with irritable bowel syndrome, headaches, and reproductive issues like impotence or infertility.

One theory behind somatization disorder is that the body has a limited capacity to cope with psychological, emotional, and social trauma. Beyond that point, the "overflow" is experienced as a physical disorder. Another theory is that such individuals have developed a heightened sensitivity to pain over time. And yet a third theory is that patients "catastrophize," or use distorted negative thinking to believe that minor ailments, like mild muscle pain or shortness of breath, are actually evidence of a serious illness such as cancer, heart disease, or a tumor.

Even though I don't consider myself prone to catastrophizing, I have definitely experienced this phenomenon myself more than once. There was one time where I developed symptoms that were very much like those of a cervical disc herniation. During a period of repeated and particularly taxing scoliosis surgeries, I experienced pain that radiated from my neck down my arm into my thumb.

I was sure I had a herniated disc and would need neck surgery. So I ordered an MRI of my spine. But there was no evidence of a herniated disc or severe nerve impingement. Eventually, I recognized that my pain was likely due, at least in part, to unconsciously shrugging my shoulders very slightly during long periods of intense concentration when the stakes were high.

Spine surgery requires a surgeon to spend hours in awkward positions to work in small areas that are tucked away in the body. I frequently tilt my neck for hours on end to decompress a nerve appropriately or insert instrumentation in less than ideal ergonomic conditions. After consideration, I noticed that when I got into those types of situations, I would actually shrug up my shoulders a bit.

Even though I saw myself as very relaxed in the operating room, I was unaware that I was tensing muscles ever so slightly, but for long periods of time. My understanding of spinal conditions, their symptoms, and distaste at the thought of requiring surgery myself made the pain grow in impact in my consciousness. Once I became aware of my overdramatic thought patterns and my poor posture—and began some specific neck exercises to strengthen the neck muscles throughout my range of motion—my pain completely went away.

While most of us engage in this type of occasional catastrophic thinking from time to time when we feel threatened or frightened, I've also encountered a number of patients with a chronic tendency to catastrophize that does not serve them well. These individuals seem to have a default pattern of negative thinking that defies any semblance of reality. When confronted with a back injury, they immediately think 17 of the most unlikely, pessimistic steps ahead, certain that the injury will cost them their job, their spouse, and their homes. While not everyone with negative thinking develops a somatization disorder, many do.

Imagine if I had continued to obsess about trying to find a cause for my neck and arm symptoms while ignoring my own psychological and physical contributions to the condition. I did, in fact, have some disc abnormalities in my neck. If pushed enough, a surgeon surely would have agreed to operate on me, especially given that my arm symptoms were identical to those of C6 nerve impingement. If I had not looked into every other cause of pain and tried multiple non-operative treatments, I could easily have undergone a surgery that would likely not have been effective.

Your Pain Is Not Imaginary

You can see the similarities here between these two schools of thought (mind-body medicine and somatic disorders). Both recognize the very real nature of pain in such cases and acknowledge the contribution from thoughts and feelings that have literally made us sick. Somatic symptoms—those painful sensations that we feel in our physical bodies—frequently occur in reaction to stressful situations. If they occur only sporadically, they aren't considered abnormal and are no cause for concern.

If you are not yet convinced about the strong connection between our emotions and pain in our bodies, look no further than headaches. It is commonly accepted that stress causes headaches. We also know that anxiety can cause constriction and pressure in the chest that can often mimic a heart attack. Also true: Strong unresolved emotions in our lives—like anger and anxiety, catastrophic thinking, and fear of the future—can manifest as chronic pain in the neck or back.

Anger is one emotion I frequently see in patients. In fact, I've noted over the years that anger is always present with chronic debilitating pain. A person may be angry at themselves because they feel they are at fault for the pain they are experiencing in some way, at someone else for hurting them, or at "the system" for not recognizing their legitimate pain by paying for medical treatment or awarding a timely settlement. Sometimes the anger is under the surface, and other times it is on display for all to see. In any case, anger is a powerful emotion that increases pain.

Another thing that alters perception of pain and other bodily sensations is anxiety. If your mind is in a state of this type of excitability, you will experience a heightened neurologic response that will cause higher perceived pain. So pain becomes much more debilitating. An area of the brain called the hippocampus is known to be important in processing pain, but is also important in learning and memory, and is part of the limbic system, which regulates emotions.

In times of immense stress or fear in both humans and other animals, this area of the brain can suppress pain transmission and perception. This important survival response can help us cope with or escape from potentially life-threatening situations. Both animal and human studies show that fear results in decreased pain reactivity, but interestingly, anxiety leads to increased pain reactivity.[6]

It is important not to label types of pain that are worsened by our mental condition as "in our head" and somehow imaginary or less valid than pain caused by an obvious physical injury like a burned hand. Quite the contrary. That would be negating a very significant aspect of how we experience pain. It's what your brain is experiencing that matters. And the severity of that pain is in large part determined by your mental and emotional state.

Narcotics, a Problematic Solution to Chronic Pain

One way to change how the brain experiences pain—whether from true physical injury or due to emotional or mental anguish—is to numb it with pain medications. For many years now, narcotics have been viewed as an effective, albeit potentially dangerous answer to pain.

Back in the late 1980s, a pivotal study was conducted by Dr. Russell Portenoy that really changed the way physicians considered and treated pain. Essentially, it concluded that pain was an untreated or undertreated condition, and that narcotics were a safe and effective long-term option for patients in pain.[7] It urged physicians to consider pain to be the fifth vital sign, after heart rate, blood pressure, temperature, and respiration rate.

As a result of that study, there was a boom in the production of synthetic drugs like OxyContin. Suddenly, these types of more potent narcotics that had been reserved for fatal diseases like cancer pain were being used casually by many with daily pain. As a result, drug overdose deaths in the United States have more than tripled since 1990. In fact, the Centers for Disease Control and Prevention reports that nearly three out of four prescription drug overdoses are caused by prescription painkillers.

> *Nearly three out of four prescription drug overdoses are caused by prescription painkillers.*

In 2008, there were 14,800 prescription painkiller deaths. And equally alarming is the fact that for every death, there were 10 treatment admissions for abuse, 32 emergency department visits, and 130 people who abuse or are dependent on painkillers. The huge rise in overdose deaths from opioids (narcotics) since 1999 parallels a 300 percent increase in their sale. Much of this can be traced back to the change in prescribing practices that came after the Portenoy study was published in 1986.

Ironically, in a 2010 interview sponsored by Physicians for Responsible Opioid Prescribing, Dr. Russell Portenoy, that study's author, expressed regret for evangelizing about opioids. He said, "To the extent that some of the adverse outcomes now are as bad as they have become in terms of endemic occurrences of addiction and unintentional overdose deaths, it's quite scary to think about how the growth in the prescribing driven by people like me led in part to that occurring."

The truth is, most patients eventually develop a tolerance to narcotics and require larger doses to get the same effect until they stop working altogether. This is why using narcotics to treat chronic pain is generally not a good idea. For many, like in the case of my patient Dave, narcotic usage can create a devastating cycle of dependency where the medication itself even *causes* an increased sensitivity to pain, the *last* thing any person wants. The mind-numbing effects of narcotics also take you away from experiencing the mind-body connection.

The good news is that in 2016 the Centers for Disease Control and Prevention released new national standards for painkillers in an attempt to tackle the growing problem of opioid medication addiction. These guidelines encourage physicians to point patients toward other methods, like over-the-counter drugs, ice, or talk therapy, before resorting to prescribing opioid medications. (And where opioids are prescribed, the CDC recommends the lowest possible dose for the shortest possible duration.)

And here's more good news: We at SpineZone have seen excellent improvement in patients' narcotics usage and their decreased reliance on prescribed medicine in general. This decreased usage occurred with medical exercise treatment alone and without any specific drug use counseling. In a sample of 121 patients who completed the program as of August 1, 2015, there was an overall 74 percent reduction in use of medications between their initial visit and their final visit.

That includes a 75 percent reduction in anti-inflammatories, a 67 percent reduction in narcotics use, and an 81 percent decrease in the use of muscle relaxants. These results are very impressive, given the debilitating conditions some of these participants arrived with. However, it also indicates that with the right protocol in place, narcotics do not need to be relied upon as heavily as many believe they do.

Chronic Pain Is Neurologically Unique

Pain is actually a useful signal since it can indicate true bodily injury. When we smash our thumb with a hammer, for example, we immediately experience an intense pain with an almost simultaneous reflex withdrawal. We then experience a delayed, lesser intense aching pain that signals some delayed inflammation and tissue damage. This type of pain is usually short-lived, or acute pain, and the inflammation and pain can be effectively treated with medication.

The longer pain goes on, however, the higher the chance that it develops into a chronic pain problem since with chronicity other factors have come into play. One main factor is the neurologic system, which can perpetuate and amplify the pain signal even without the presence of tissue damage, creating a pain pathway that becomes the problem in and of itself. In this case, pain is the disease rather than the symptoms of an injury.

The way the person thinks about the pain, as we discussed earlier, as well as emotional states such as anxiety and depression, are other factors that can affect the perception of pain. Other factors include lack of exercise or physical deconditioning, which we will address in later chapters.

The way our brains perceive chronic pain is particularly unique. In fact, researchers have studied chronic pain by watching which areas of the brain light up on a functional MRI. The fMRI, as we discussed earlier, measures brain activity by identifying changes in blood flow in various parts of the brain, where there are more metabolic activities.

What researchers find is that for patients suffering from chronic pain, many areas of the brain become involved in processing pain, compared to far fewer areas of the brain when processing a trauma that causes a singular episode of pain. When we experience a painful stimulus in the arm, for example, it is transmitted to the spinal cord, and then relayed up to the midbrain and terminates at the primary sensory area of the brain. The primary somatosensory cortex, as it is called, contains essentially a map with a direct representation of the body on it.

All sensory input lands there, but then gets "interpreted" by different areas of the brain. However, in patients with chronic pain, it is as if there is an avalanche of brain activity that occurs downstream of the somatosensory cortex. This avalanche includes a complex biochemical pathway of inflammation that spreads to many areas of the brain. Additionally, there is a psychosocial circuit that spreads to even further areas of the brain.

It is thought that the mechanisms activated when animals and humans are in chronic pain are similar to those that are activated when they are sick. There is an inflammatory cascade that results in the body being rendered more inactive and dormant to facilitate recovery. Functionally, chronic pain can induce an inflammatory process that increases pain awareness and sensitization to limit further injury.[8] This makes sense when we consider that patients with chronic pain have a profound lack of motivation for activity that is disproportionate to their level of injury.

If you go to the dentist with tooth pain, you will likely get a specific diagnosis of an abnormality in a certain tooth that corresponds with your pain. Yet, when it comes to chronic lower back pain, we know the exact diagnosis less than 20 percent of the time. Chronic pain is not like the kind of pain you feel when you bang your hand with a hammer. It's much more complex than that and requires a deeper analysis.

My Own Experience Brings About an Effective Treatment

A number of years ago, early in my practice, several factors converged in my life that substantially increased my sense of stress. In my professional life, I was working through some challenges with my partner and I was unsure which way things would go. Personally, my wife was lobbying to move back to her native New York from San Diego, which was not part of my plan. To me, it felt like all the foundations I had carefully built over the years were in jeopardy. It was a very difficult time for me, one that was full of uncertainty.

As an ambitious and focused individual, I was frustrated that things were not going as planned. I started to notice that I was less patient and easily irritated. At the urging of a good friend of mine who himself had a life-changing experience, I decided to attend a Vipassana retreat near Yosemite to learn how to better accept all the uncertainty in my life.

"Vipassana," which means "to see things as they really are," is a 2,500-year-old Indian tradition of meditation that was long lost to humanity and then rediscovered. It is a process of self-purification and self-observation as a "universal remedy for universal ills." To learn the technique, participants attend a ten-day residential course where they meditate 15 to 18 hours a day in silence.

Since the purpose of learning this meditation technique is to practice being "non-reactive," the evening before each day of meditation begins with a one-hour talk from a teacher who provides wonderfully colorful vignettes that illustrate how out of control our minds get with worry and expectations. He then outlines the meditation instructions to be followed the next day.

The first three days involve only mastering concentration and quieting the mind, which takes some practice. If you have never tried this, attempt to sit quietly without having any thoughts. Not more than 15 or 20 seconds will pass until a thought will intrude upon this silence. This barrage of often unwanted thoughts forms the basis for much of what ails us, yet it is impossible to forcefully stop the bombardment.

After those three days, however, we were able to use this newly found focus of our mind to scan our bodies, sensing whatever sensation was there at the moment. He said that our strong reactions, whether they are aversions *to* things or strong cravings *for* things essentially make us crazy; that instead of labeling things "good" or "bad," it's important to just accept how things are.

He explained that reactions create a disturbance in the body. Let's liken it to a line being drawn. This line can create a ripple on the surface of one's being that dissipates naturally, like a line in the sand that is washed away by an ocean wave. The problem is that the line that we create can also be memorialized in cement and create a deep and permanent scar that resurfaces in unwanted ways.

Our thoughts can therefore have a profound physical impact on our bodies when we allow them to race, or conversely, when we react and repress them. He urged us to experience our feelings fully without reaction so they could wash away without a physical manifestation. Through Vipassana meditation, I learned that when I would bury a feeling or reaction, I'd really just push it deeper and strengthen it, empowering it to manifest later.

During my 10 days of meditation, I personally experienced the way the body memorializes emotional pain through physical sensations. Before the retreat, I hadn't connected the stressors in my life to the strange sensations I had been experiencing below my collarbone. But during meditation, when I scanned my body and came upon the sensation in my collarbone, it would re-ignite all of the specific anger and disappointment in my current situation, ripe with emotions and memories that I thought I had already forgotten.

However, with the teachings, I observed that the sensations would arise spontaneously and then resolve, and the less I reacted to the sensation in my collarbone, the less strongly I felt about the anger and disappointment in my situation. I truly saw how bodily sensations were connected with unresolved emotions.

After the retreat, I noticed that those anxious, often angry, and disappointed emotions left, permanently. I was able to better relate to my wife and understand her point of view, and arrived at an amicable solution with my partner. I found that I could also finally let go of the disappointment about my knee (and my athletic aspirations) as well as my expectations about my future.

During the retreat, I had stopped reacting to the sinking, stuck-in-quicksand feeling I experienced when scanning near my knee. After the retreat and to this day, I enjoy whatever tennis brings me, from playing mixed doubles tournaments with my daughter to even warming up my kids for their tournaments. This has also helped ensure that any feelings I had about my own unrealized potential do not manifest in anxiety over my kids' athletics.

After returning to my spine practice, I identified many other ways that our emotions and bodily sensations are intertwined. When it comes to the spine and the neck, most people consider this structure to be their core, foundational to their bodies. As a result, it's commonplace to hold emotional pain there, just as it is in the area near the heart, where I experienced discomfort and even shortness of breath. (Or near the eyes also, as I recall one of the retreat participants talked about. She acknowledged her struggle with worrying about how others perceived her.)

I understood that things manifested the way they were meant to manifest. I believe that over a lifetime, certain "weaknesses" in our character express themselves in circumstances in our lives. We either accept and learn from these experiences, or fight them and react, which can often cause emotional pain. In my case, it was my ambitious, narrow focus about how I expected my life to unfold.

Vipassana meditation taught me how to accept and embrace what *is* so that I feel my emotions fully and avoid letting them become trapped in my body. This doesn't mean you should surrender to your circumstance or avoid trying to shape your destiny; rather, it actually frees you to use your imagination and all of your power to shape your life!

I left that retreat with a deep sense of serenity. By better learning how to "ride the wave" of whatever was going on, I reacted less to the inevitable events in life. Now I have a skill (meditation) that I can turn to even for 15 minutes at a time to maintain a sense of deep calm and purpose.

Vipassana may or may not be for you. I share it here with you only as an example of a powerful tool that I experienced personally in a deep way, which helped shape my understanding of how we hold emotional pain in our bodies and how we can resolve it. While I had read about psychological pain and its manifestations many times in the medical literature before the retreat, I found that I gained a true appreciation of its significance only after experiencing it for myself. There are plenty of other excellent ways you can learn to disconnect from feelings that are overwhelming your body. The important thing is that you find a way that works for you to address any emotional components of pain you may be experiencing.

THE BASICS OF MEDITATION

The prospect of meditating can be daunting for the beginner or uninitiated, but it is actually much easier than you may think. The benefits of meditation, which will help you strengthen your intuitive faculties, far outweigh the effort to add this to your daily ablutions. By quieting the incessant mental chatter in your mind, you will uncover your own truths.

There are many schools of thought regarding meditation. As mentioned, I spent a sizable amount of time learning and practicing Vipassana, so I am best suited to discuss that technique. But I must preface my comments by declaring that I am not a trained meditation instructor. Nonetheless, I am such a believer in meditation's spiritual and physical benefits, that if I could make a small difference in encouraging interest in this practice, I would feel a true sense of accomplishment. Below are the basics of what I have learned.

First sit in a comfortable position. If your hips and knees are healthy, it's best to sit cross-legged on the ground, with a small pillow placed behind your buttock. Otherwise sit in a chair with proper posture (See figure in Chapter 2). I find it less effective to meditate lying down since it is very easy to fall asleep.

Now, focus on your breath. Feel its warmth as you exhale and notice the relatively cooler breath when you inhale. Sense the rhythm of the breath, the length of exhalation versus inhalation. Concentrate on the small area around your nostrils for any sensation that may arise. You will invariably notice an intruding thought arise within 15-30 seconds. Don't react; simply refocus on the breath. Eventually, you will get better at this and extend your thought-free intervals.

The breath is a great bridge between the conscious and subconscious. We can voluntarily alter our breath speed and depth, yet when we don't think about it, the breath continues involuntarily. It automatically varies based on our thoughts, speeding up when we are anxious and slowing as we relax. Sense your breath's character. Notice how it changes when thoughts arise depending on the emotion associated with the thought.

Practice this technique for 10 minutes each day, focusing only on the breath and quieting the mind. Do this for at least a week and notice whether it becomes easier over time. The goal is to eventually be able to meditate for a minimum of 15-20 minutes a day.

After this initial week, you have likely built an improved focus that will serve you well as you scan your body for subtle sensations. I still like to begin every meditation session with a few minutes of focused breathing, then transition to scanning the body. Slowly move up your body, starting with your toes. Take note of anything you are feeling, no matter how insignificant. Don't shy away from unpleasant or painful sensations, but also be sure you don't give them more attention than any other area of your body. The goal is to foster a sense of equanimity, or complete non-reactivity, and acceptance of the way things are, not the way we wish them to be.

This is a simplification, but our suffering often arises from us not accepting life the way it is. We tend to crave experiences that we consider desirable and feel aversion to the undesirable. Every life event can either be accepted and just pass through us, or leave a scar when we react in anger or fear. The deeper the reaction, the deeper the scar. This meditative practice stops the creation of any further scars and can help clear up old ones.

For this reason, meditation is an incredibly powerful tool. When our mind is out of control, reeling over worst-case scenarios, meditation has the power to quietly dissolve these thoughts. When any sensation, including pain, starts to take hold of our function and life, we could all use the ability to dispassionately observe the pain as it melts away.

I would encourage anyone who feels inclined to delve deeper into Vipassana to listen to the discourses available at www.dhamma.org. Or better yet, attend one of the 10-day retreats held in over 170 international centers (see website for details). They are free of charge (they do ask for a donation of any amount you wish) and truly transformational.

The Personal Motivation Factor

We have discussed how meditation can quiet the mind and address the underlying emotional causes of pain. Now we will cover another tool you can use to combat pain: motivation. Yes, for many people, the ability to overcome pain or at least live productively with it comes down to how badly they want to do so.

Juan was a 38-year-old construction worker whose foot broke through a plank that was temporarily placed over a large pothole. As a result of his foot unexpectedly sinking, he twisted his back and sustained a significant disc herniation in his lower back, which resulted in sciatica.

I treated him by prescribing an epidural injection and physical therapy. He improved somewhat, but still had significant leg pain with only very minimal weakness and numbness. I had not cleared him to return back to work due to his persistent and noteworthy symptoms. However, he had two small children at home. I began to see that his fear of losing his job and loss of income were starting to wear on his sensibilities as the breadwinner of the family.

About four months after the injury, he returned to the office for a follow-up visit where I discussed his treatment options with him. My opinion was that he met the classical indications for a person who would benefit from discectomy surgery, which would truly improve his pain. I explained the surgery to him in detail, as well as the post-operative course, which included about six weeks of healing before beginning physical therapy as well as another six to twelve weeks before he could return to his regular, physically demanding job.

Juan desperately wanted to go back to work. He asked me what would happen if he elected to forgo the surgery. I told him that disc herniations often spontaneously resolve in the first three months after onset, but generally if they don't improve within that first three- to six-month period, the pain would likely continue for years, but could still resolve gradually over time. Since he was not significantly weak or numb, there was no real risk of long-term neurologic damage.

After much discussion and deliberation with his family, Juan returned and asked me to release him back to work, informing me that he didn't want to proceed with surgery. He said that when he looked at his children's faces, he knew he had the strength to tolerate the pain and continue to work and earn for them. While work was difficult for him at first, he did find that he was gradually able to tolerate it better and better.

Juan's story is a great example of how our perception of pain changes greatly depending on our motivations. In fact, it's clearly documented in the medical literature. I've seen in many, many patients how motivations can work both for and against a person. In the case of patients who feel victimized—perhaps because they were hit in a car accident or have filed a workers' compensation claim due to an injury sustained at work—they frequently experience more pain and do not respond as well to treatment as others.

In the case of such claims, an individual typically receives a higher settlement if he or she is more impaired. And rightly so. But here is the problem: Even though the vast majority of these patients do not consciously intend to deceive anyone, some patients have a strong focus on how poorly they are doing. This pessimistic view along with the urge to convince others of their dire status seriously impedes their recovery, not just with back disorders, but also with painful upper extremity overuse injuries.

Because these patients don't have a sense of control about their futures, they are frequently angry. They may feel they are at the mercy of their insurance company with regard to authorizing care they feel they need. The anger and powerlessness create even more psychological pain.

And as a result, it's well documented that such individuals are among the biggest consumers of healthcare and also have the poorest outcomes.[9] When I see such patients, I frequently counsel them to bring this awareness to their situation. I inform them that if they prolong the fighting without good medical justification for more of a settlement, they may obtain bigger compensation, but this will likely take a long time and may not be worth it overall, especially if they lose their job and stop working altogether. I urge them to continue to pursue the settlement they deserve, but—and here is an important difference—without attachment to the outcome.

Is Self-Victimization Worth the Cost?

Is it really worth gaining a few extra thousand dollars in a settlement if it means you may not recover your health, sense of well-being, or work again? (It is a well-known fact that in workers' compensation cases, patients who do not return to work within two years are unlikely to ever do so. Furthermore, there is just a 50 percent chance that an injured employee will return to work after a six-month absence.[10])

Is it worth permanent disability to remain steadfastly determined to show how injured and helpless you are? Time and again, I see such patients three or five years after our initial visit, and they are much, much worse. It is toxic to live with negative feelings for so long. They find their way into your body.

The goal is to live in the moment. A settlement claim will not go more quickly when the patient remains angry, anxious, and worried about the outcome. The system is what it is, so I urge patients not to give away their power. Rather, empower yourself—take back control—by investing your energy in healing now rather than in how the lawsuit turns out later. Negative thinking and anxiety about the future will hurt your ability to recover.

Conversely, I have also met many patients, like Juan, who have overcome severe pain through a strong positive motivator. They provide another great example of how even severe structural deficits that we can see on an MRI don't necessarily require surgery.

The pain that we feel depends on the brain's perception of it. If someone is filled with love and caring (perhaps they are the daily caregiver of a grandchild or the breadwinner of a busy household), their body produces hormones like oxytocin that allow them to tolerate pain better. They may also unconsciously minimize the pain they experience because they feel a higher responsibility. As a result, they are more resilient than we would expect them to be.

So in summary, I urge you to think a bit about your own emotional life and its potential role in any back pain you may be experiencing. Are you feeling anxious, angry, or stressed? Don't underestimate the powerful role those emotions play. Are you someone who tends to catastrophize or focus a great deal on physical sensations in your body? If so, you're not alone. The good news is that there are many approaches to addressing these drivers of pain so you can regain a sense of control and power in your life...and put pain behind you.

Key Learning Points: Suffering Lies Within

1. Thoughts and anxiety manifest as physical symptoms in our bodies.
2. We experience pain through a complex interplay between our minds and our bodies.
3. Pain is not imaginary. Just because our thoughts and feelings contribute to our perception of pain, these types of pain cannot be discounted as "in our head." It's what your brain is experiencing that matters.
4. Chronic pain is unique because it creates an avalanche of activity in many areas of the brain and even inflammation that is similar to when we are sick. As a result, it is more complex to treat.

5. Personal motivation—for better or for worse—plays
   an important role in our recovery from back pain.

CHAPTER 4

TREATING THE WHOLE PERSON

> "Do not dwell in the past; do not dream of the future; concentrate the mind on the present moment."
>
> —Buddha

There are many practices you can use to successfully shift your emotional reality if your goal is to take back control of your life from pain. And the wonderful thing about the process is that you will likely find that your work in this area spills over into many other areas of life to create a positive effect in your relationships, work, and leisure activities. It can truly be transformative.

I want you to fully realize that managing your back pain often requires a "whole person" approach to healing. In other words, your mindset matters just as much as your physical condition (and, in fact, the two cannot be separated). Whether your pain comes from a work or sports injury or age-related degeneration, your point of view regarding your physical limitations can make all the difference in the world when it comes to pursuing wellness.

If you allow yourself to stew in anger, misery, woe, or helplessness, I promise, your journey will be harder than it needs to be. Your thoughts and attitudes will make a difference in how you feel, and therefore they are just as important in your recovery as your medical treatments. What's more, the decisions you make should take into account your whole life circumstance—what you need to be able to do for your job, which hobbies you can't live without, and so forth. (This is another facet of the "whole person" approach.)

If you stay positive and focused on your current state and take every possible step to improve your physical and emotional condition, your healing will come more easily and more naturally. But if you allow yourself to wallow in negativity, then your journey will be far less pleasant.

In other words, your perspective will absolutely influence your healing, and a healthy emotional state is a crucial step in treating your whole self.

Nancy's Story: How Catastrophizing Makes Things Worse

We talked about catastrophizing pain in Chapter 3. Catastrophic thinking is a dangerous practice—and yet so many of us do it daily, whether or not we face pain. Have you ever received a cryptic email from your boss requesting a meeting and immediately decide you are being fired or downsized? So often we let our wild imaginations override logic and common sense in this way. Catastrophizing is a bad habit that most of us could stand to live without. It wastes our energy, leaves us upset and disempowered, and we make unwise decisions based upon it.

When it comes to back pain—in fact, any aspect of health—it's common for patients to catastrophize by magnifying the negatives. "I have this pain in my leg," an individual might say, but then magnify the fears to, "I just know I'm going to get weaker and weaker until I'm bedbound!" Or:"I have this bad disc disease that will continue to cause me worsening pain. If I don't have surgery to fix it right now, I'm going to end up in a wheelchair!"

> *When it comes to back pain—in fact,*
> *any aspect of health—it's common for*
> *patients to catastrophize by magnify-*
> *ing the negatives.*

In the same way, people tend to minimize the positives. "I saw three surgeons for an opinion on my back pain," such a person might say. "But only one of them said I could probably get better without surgery. Only *one* of them!"Yet a person who had learned to focus on positive possibilities would likely be thrilled to know there was hope for a non-operative solution.

Sometimes, despite strong evidence to the contrary, we still cling to our strong negative thoughts. That's how significantly they affect us. Many years ago, I saw a patient in her late 20s, Nancy, whose story has always stayed with me as a cautionary tale about giving in to our negative thinking.

While Nancy was attractive and slim, she didn't actively exercise. So it was perhaps not surprising that working in a sedentary and high-intensity customer service job took a toll on her body. Besides her lack of exercise and the inherent stress of dealing with unhappy customers—both of which can contribute to pain— Nancy made many repetitive movements throughout her workday. From her desk and computer, she was constantly contorting her body to look over her left and right shoulders at customers.

Eventually, she developed pain in her neck as well as severe arm pain, including some numbness and weakness. She was very scared as she'd never had a serious illness and considered herself to be a very healthy person. She wanted to be diligent in addressing and fixing her problem, though, so she immediately saw an orthopedic surgeon who diagnosed a disc herniation in her neck based on an MRI. He told her it would likely eventually require surgery.

At that point, even though it had been only 10 days since she'd first experienced the pain, she became very focused on the size of her disc herniation and the anticipated need for this surgery. But because it is very common for disc issues like these to resolve on their own if given a little time to heal, the surgeon recommended she wait on surgery and begin some physical therapy.

Refusing to heed the surgeon's advice, Nancy kept pressing him to do the surgery. In her mind, once it was discussed as a cure, surgery was the only way her problem would go away. While she did start some physical therapy, she later admitted to me that she participated less than wholeheartedly and quit early since she didn't believe it would really work.

When she saw me four weeks after the injury for a second opinion, I concurred with the surgeon that despite the herniation, it was important to wait on surgery. Even more to the point, by objective measures, the numbness and weakness had become milder and it did not appear to be a progressive problem.

But Nancy couldn't let go of the fact that she felt she needed this surgery to cure her problem. So five weeks after the onset of symptoms, the surgeon succumbed to her insistence and obliged her by removing and fusing her disc. I wouldn't see her next until 18 months later at which point she would come back to see me because she was *still in pain*.

To surgically treat disc herniations in the neck, the disc is completely removed. The remaining space is filled with bone to allow the body to grow new bone and fuse or "weld" the disc space, and often screws and plates are inserted in order to hold the vertebrae in position until the fusion occurs. In Nancy's case, the bone fusion didn't take, meaning that the body was not able to grow bone to weld the disc space together. (This can happen despite optimal conditions.)

And so she underwent another surgery nine months later. By that time, she'd had a second MRI that showed the disc above the problem disc was also degenerated, and so the surgeon set out to fix both issues with a second surgery aimed at fusing two discs.

However, when the surgeon inserted the bone screw in surgery number two, it went a bit askew and violated the normal disc above it. By the time Nancy saw me six months after that second surgery, a new MRI showed that due to irritation from the screw placed in the disc, the upper disc was prematurely deteriorated.

The surgeon was recommending yet a third operation. By now, she had had two surgeries and was facing a third surgery and three-level fusion. (The more discs a person has fused, the lower the success rate and the higher the likelihood that the next disc up will deteriorate and, if operated upon, not fuse properly.) Nancy, unfortunately, ended up going through with the third surgery.

Nancy's case really stuck with me. I was saddened by her unfortunate experience. Despite some improvement after sustaining her initial disc herniation, she decided to still pursue the surgery—which set her on this path of multiple unsuccessful operations.

Cervical disc surgery is one of our most successful surgeries, yet it still needs to be employed at the right time and for the right patient. There is an almost 95 percent success rate with a one-level fusion.[1] Instrumentation-related complications occur less than 0.1 percent of the time.[2] The increased risk of adjacent disc degeneration is low but well documented.[3] Unfortunately, Nancy was one of the unlucky ones who experienced problem after problem once she decided to pursue surgery rather than wait.

When I last left off with Nancy, she was just 31 and had undergone three surgeries and had three fused discs, with no good solutions in the future to address her now chronic pain.

I wonder what would have happened in Nancy's case if the findings on the MRI scan were discussed, but minimized, by emphasizing the studies that show how well patients with disc herniations can do with non-operative treatment. In fact, many studies show that even massive disc herniations can fully reabsorb by doing nothing in particular, and patients can have great long-term outcomes.[4,5]

> *Many studies show that even massive*
> *disc herniations can fully reabsorb.*

Cases like Nancy's emphasize how catastrophic thinking—instead of thoughtfully considering all treatment options—can sometimes lead to lasting negative results.

Steve's Story: Why You Shouldn't Fixate on MRI Results

Even after initially focusing on the MRI, patients will reluctantly, and with coaxing, accept an alternative course of treatment—as long as the surgeon recommending this course shows confidence that the patient will do well without surgery. But it still surprises me how difficult it is for patients to let go of their need to fix what they see on a diagnostic study…even if that's not really causing the problem.

Steve was one such case. He was an avid 49-year-old cyclist who wanted to get my opinion on surgery for a herniated disc that had been recommended to him. He had developed very severe back pain that had radiated to his buttocks and legs. Steve explained that the pain had been so incapacitating that he couldn't work for a week. After that first week, his pain improved and was now gone, except for a persistent "foot drop." In other words, his foot would sort of flop whenever he took a step and this was also interfering with his cycling hob-by.

Steve had seen a spine surgeon two weeks after the onset of pain who had strongly advised surgery to re-lieve nerve pressure after identifying a large disc herni-ation on his MRI scan. Then he saw a different surgeon for a second opinion a week later who had told him that since he had no pain, he did not recommend the surgery solely for the weakness in his foot. Since he had been prepared to have the surgery, this second opinion just floored him.

When Steve asked me which surgeon I agreed with, I said that since he was pain-free, I was inclined to agree with the second one. This prompted me to order a neu-rologic study called a "nerve conduction and EMG" to get a baseline on nerve function so we could determine if it was recovering over time. The results shocked me. The nerve study showed the abnormality was actually coming from the peroneal nerve that comes around the fibula—the small bone on the outside of the *knee*—and not the nerve from the *back*.

How is this possible? Think of the nerves connect-ing the head to the legs as electrical wiring. There are multiple "circuit breakers" that are vulnerable and can become tripped along the way, causing foot drop. The most common area for the fuse to be tripped is as the nerves pass by disc herniations in the back.

But another much less likely cause can be when the wire passes along the outside of the knee. Even though the most common cause of foot drop is compression of the spinal nerve by a disc herniation, Steve's foot drop was more likely due to a rare abnormality of the nerve at the knee.

The neurologist who performed the nerve study and I both agreed that the problem Steve was experiencing was likely not related to the disc issue seen on the MRI. It was clearly coming from the diminished function of the nerve crossing at the knee. And yet, Steve still pushed for the surgery. "I'm really worried about this disc causing pressure on my nerve," he said. "Shouldn't I just go ahead and do the surgery to relieve the pressure we see on the MRI?"

So instead of relief that his problem was not back related, and in spite of clear evidence that the problem was likely due to another problem, Steve still felt compelled by the "objectivity" of the MRI showing the disc compressing on his nerve. Sure enough, when I saw him 10 weeks later, he reported that his foot strength had improved a great deal. And yet, he asked me one more time, "Shouldn't we just take out that disc?" (Of course not!) In fact, he even paid cash for a second MRI, which showed no change in the size of the disc. These two cases illustrate the fallacy of a common and prevalent myth...that if you have a significant abnormality on a spine MRI scan, you need surgery to address it.

> *It's a myth that if you have a terrible-looking MRI scan, you need surgery.*

In fact, there are far more patients walking around with abnormal findings on MRIs that don't need treatment than there are patients with those same abnormal findings that *do* need treatment or surgery. In stark contrast to other types of studies that are truly diagnostic of an abnormality that needs to be addressed, many abnormal MRI findings in the spine can frequently be safely ignored clinically if they do not correlate with a patient's complaints or physical examination findings.

This is why it is so important that we don't allow our overly analytical minds to fool us into clinging to ideas that don't make sense scientifically or push for treatment we don't need. It's not that MRIs are unnecessary; in fact, they are incredibly useful. They need to be used judiciously, however, and the diagnostic findings need to be placed into perspective. Not everybody with a back problem needs an MRI, and not everybody with abnormalities on the MRI has an actual problem.

> *Not everybody with a back problem needs an MRI, and not everybody with abnormalities on the MRI has an actual problem.*

It is a very human tendency to jump to the worst conclusion and let the "what ifs" drive decisions. Even though "worst-case scenario thinking" doesn't show up on an MRI scan, it must also be acknowledged and treated by appropriate counseling as to the meaning of the MRI findings, and as another step in addressing pain. The spine is an important part of the body, but so is the mind, with its tremendous power over how we view and approach health challenges.

As we've seen through the examples of Nancy and Steve, even the most intelligent among us can benefit from tools to replace errors in thinking with more rational thoughts to stop our out-of-control, unfounded fears. But can we really change this tendency to let our minds run away with us? The answer is a definitive yes.

Breaking the Thought Cycle Through Cognitive Behavioral Therapy

One of the most recognized therapeutic approaches for effectively treating chronic pain is called "cognitive behavioral therapy" or CBT. "Cognitive" refers to recognizing the negative thoughts and feelings that occur when you have back pain. "Behavioral" refers to learning how to change the cognitive negativity into healthy thoughts and actions. It's a form of psychotherapy that focuses on creating awareness of inaccurate or negative patterns of behavior that are common in patients with chronic low back pain.

These thoughts typically include ideas like, *I will never be able to rid myself of back pain, I will need surgery for sure*, or *I will never be able to play golf again*. Cognitive behavioral approaches replace these errors in thinking with more positive and rational thoughts such as, *My disc can repair itself once I gradually strengthen my back* or *With patience and hard work, I will return to the sports I love*. As a result, an individual gains insight into how to better respond to difficult situations. By challenging irrational beliefs, we can help a patient reduce emotional distress and self-defeating behavior.

CBT is very effective for a wide range of mental health issues that range from depression and anxiety to eating and sleep disorders. Studies also show that CBT is effective for treating patients with chronic lower back pain because it can address the psychological component of the pain, whether that is anger, grief, divorce, or isolation.[6,7] Unlike other types of talk therapy that may require years to achieve a meaningful breakthrough,

CBT is typically effective in several months of focused work.

By personally experiencing the capabilities of the body and even borrowing from some of CBT's fundamental principles, we can apply and adapt them for an effective back treatment plan. For example, in CBT therapy, patients begin by first reporting on a series of measures to determine how impaired their thinking is so the therapist can identify how best to treat it. Then with the therapist, the patient learns how to challenge irrational thoughts that have been identified.

Over the years, I have found that most of the irrational thoughts in patients with chronic back pain are centered around their loss of function. They often foster a distorted view of their body's capabilities due to their previous experiences of pain and their perceived limitations based on their back condition. Their challenge is to fight back against this tendency and treat their damaged thoughts in the same way they hope to rehabilitate their damaged bodies.

Patients undergoing CBT acquire new skills to deal with the daily challenges they face so they can break the cycle of these automatic thoughts, substituting new skills that are gradually "hardwired." Homework, a hallmark of CBT, reinforces the new skills they are learning. Near the end of treatment, patients identify coping skills for the future and may follow-up in post-treatment assessments so the therapist can evaluate how well they are applying their new skills in daily living.[8]

I am sure you know of many examples in your own life or the lives of others where new coping skills have overcome poor thinking. Perhaps you conquered your fear of computers by perfecting one skill at a time, until your proficiency improved to the point where your fear went away. By using this same principle at SpineZone, we have noted miraculous improvements in both function and attitude that have resulted from experiencing motion and realizing strength.

You can use these same principles, even though it can be challenging when you must overcome years of entrenched negative thinking or circumstances. Begin by seeking knowledge from reliable sources and doing what you can in a stepwise and deliberate fashion. Also, try to view your negative beliefs as hypotheses rather than facts. Test them out by "running experiments." In other words, find out if they are actually true by challenging them.

To get you started on the road toward recovery, I have a homework assignment just for you. Below I have listed several affirmations that you can use daily in order to start hardwiring your thoughts for healing and success. Remember how inextricably linked your thoughts are to how you view your health journey. This guidance will help you begin to gently shift your perspective to a more positive place.

HEALING AFFIRMATIONS

1. **Limiting thought:** My MRI scan shows multiple abnormalities. I will always have pain and be limited.
   Affirmation: My MRI results don't doom me to suffering. In fact, most people develop

significant abnormalities on their MRI without ever having any symptoms.

2. **Limiting thought:** My injury is so severe I am sure I will never work again.

   Affirmation: I am taking it day by day and choose to acknowledge my progress.

3. **Limiting thought:** I have degenerative disc "disease." No wonder I need to restrict what I can do.

   Affirmation: Degenerative disc disease is not a disease at all and shouldn't affect my happiness. It's like wrinkles; we all get them as we age and how we perceive them defines their effect on our lives.

4. **Limiting thought:** I am sure my partner/family/friends will abandon me.

   Affirmation: I have a support system of people who love and support me on my journey to wellness.

5. **Limiting thought:** This is the worst thing that has ever happened to me.

   Affirmation: This injury does not define who I am. I am more than this pain and have lots of good things in my life.

6. **Limiting thought:** I can't handle this much pain.

   Affirmation: I am still here. I am overcoming this obstacle right now, and by observing yet not reacting to it, I am taking away its power over me.

7. **Limiting thought:** I don't have time to commit to recovery!

   Affirmation: I am lovingly giving my body the time and resources it needs to heal.

8. **Limiting thought:** I will never be as fit and strong as I once was—and there's nothing I can do about it.

   Affirmation: My body knows how to heal, and I am willing to help it day by day.

The SpineZone Approach Targets Mind AND Body (and Helps Patients Face Their Pain)

Just as a certified cognitive behavioral therapist may be necessary to help us think differently when we can't extricate ourselves from our thoughts, you may need to seek the help of experienced practitioners who can isolate your back joints and muscles to improve your range of motion and strength without causing pain or more damage. Since the mind-body connection is so strong, you can improve your condition by working on either the mind or the body or both together.

This is an important concept. By the time pain has taken a foothold in your life, it is sometimes difficult to know where to start for concrete gains—especially when it comes to the mind. This is why for most of us, it is more challenging to deal with the psychological aspects that contribute to our pain than to take incremental steps and connect with our bodies directly.

It is more challenging to deal with the psychological aspects that contribute to our pain than to take incremental steps and connect with our bodies directly.

In our SpineZone clinics, instead of focusing on the limiting thoughts themselves, we take patients through specialized exercises that allow them to experience what their bodies can actually *do*. By isolating the muscles, we take pressure off of the joints so that the spine can actually start to move and the muscles can start to fire again. When patients experience this breakthrough firsthand, the catastrophic thoughts go away because they actually see that progress is possible.

Patients who have suffered injury to their spines are often scared and traumatized. And it really is no wonder. An injury such as a herniated disc can indeed affect a person's whole life for a significant period of time. Disc problems can be recurrent, resulting in years of oscillating pain, progressive weakness, an alarming fear of activity, and a precipitous decline in function. The emotional component crescendos to the point of overriding the rational mind and resulting in a fixation on the avoidance of pain. The method of treatment at SpineZone clinics takes this important factor in patients' psyches into account so that we are helping the patients reach emotional healing as well as physical.

Post-traumatic stress disorder is an extreme example of a mental health disorder that results when the "thinking part" of the brain (the frontal lobes) and the "feeling part" of the brain (the limbic system) don't talk to each other effectively. When some individuals with PTSD experience traumatic events (e.g., warfare, sexual assault, serious injury), they may relive these fearful experiences over and over again even though they are no longer occurring. They may be triggered by a sharp noise or vision due to an overactive amygdala in the brain.

In her book *Train Your Mind, Change Your Brain*, author Sharon Begley explains how in one study, people with PTSD underwent a specialized and related type of treatment called "exposure and response therapy" to find relief. She explains that they were repeatedly exposed to the trigger (i.e., a noise) in a safe and comfortable setting and eventually no longer responded with anxiety. This is because the amygdala, the region of the brain that is overactive and creates fear in people who suffer from PTSD, quieted down.

In other words, those thinking regions of the brain send inhibitory connections to the amygdala to calm it. Exposure and response therapy is also effective for treating obsessive-compulsive disorder and phobias. Interestingly, it turns out that when we actively try to avoid something—like an unpleasant thought—we really just "charge" that thought and give it more power.

> *When we actively try to avoid something—like an unpleasant thought—we really just give it more power.*

At SpineZone, we essentially do our own version of exposure therapy. By repeatedly "exposing" patients to their spinal condition and their perceived lack of function through conditioning exercises, they learn to "face the fear and do it anyway." There is a cognitive dissonance that must resolve when their irrational fears are shown to be just that. Even though they may be fearful in the beginning because they are in pain, they see over time—through their own experience doing customized exercises—that these fears are irrational as their pain resolves and their strength improves. Furthermore, they are able to see that they, in fact, can still function even though they may remain in some pain.

In fact, these kinds of results are borne out by studies that have looked at PET scans of the brains of people who have undergone exposure and response therapy. The scans show that these repeated and planned exposures have actually rewired their brains so that those limiting thoughts lose their power; they no longer create fear and anxiety in us.[9]

By my own experience, I have noted that this realistic approach works well. When the SpineZone team evaluates and formulates a treatment program for a patient, they begin by understanding the patient's perception of their problem and what their goals are. Then they perform a physical examination, and if diagnostic tests are available (and especially if the patient is focused on them), they are reviewed.

During their course of treatment, we try to stick to as many objective parameters as we can, such as measuring the patient's strength and range of motion, and then following their progress throughout treatment. When need be, the appropriate practitioner is used to address specific concerns.

For example, if the patient is focused on their need for surgery, who better than a surgeon who also has experience with our training methods, successes, and limitations to address that concern? It is only by treating the whole person—understanding how they need to move at work and at play—that we can design an effective program to maximize an individual's potential.

Fortunately, I was able to convince Steve not to have unnecessary surgery just because he was focused on the abnormal MRI. However, Nancy did not have enough patience to wait. I am convinced that with the progress she was making, her initial disc herniation had a high probability of resolving, and with the appropriate therapy she would have been fully functional with, at most, only occasional neck pain. While neither Steve nor Nancy were impaired enough to be referred for CBT in the early stages of symptoms, they both could have clearly benefited from applying some of these tools to their thought processes.

A Whole-Person Approach Is the Intuitive and Obvious Solution

I am not a psychologist or psychiatrist and don't consider myself to be an expert in these fields. However, I realize that I have consciously and unconsciously used many of these techniques for years with my patients. Like it or not, we each use many of these approaches in our daily lives to influence others. (When trying to convince others of erroneous thoughts, we often quote an expert or refer to a person's direct experiences that contradict an irrational belief.)

As an expert in the spine surgery field, I'm in a unique position to help create awareness about inaccurate thoughts regarding surgery and to offer perspective on its necessity and timing. By being intricately involved in the actual rehabilitation, I can bring that experience to bear and provide credible alternatives to those who have concerns about pursuing rehabilitation due to significant abnormalities on their diagnostic studies.

I find that patients respond best when they actually *experience* success for themselves, rather than just hearing about how to attain it. When appropriate, a combination of advice and experience works best. Patients need to feel confident that their specific condition can be helped without surgery, and then they need to experience actual changes through spine therapy exercises.

> *Patients respond best when they actually* experience *success, rather than just hearing about it.*

For us, that has been achieved best in an integrated model that includes the spine surgeon and staff with the therapists. It's inspiring to note the before and after differences in a patient after four to six weeks of training…not just in their reduction of pain, but also in their mental outlook and confidence.

Your Future Life Trajectory—and How It Should Affect Your Decision Making

I am all about maximizing the body's function at every stage of life, and in fact, much of this book is devoted to that end. However, regardless of what the path to recovery may be, it bears mentioning at this point how important it is to have realistic expectations, *even while* aiming high for an optimal recovery.

I am often faced with patients who wish to undergo spine surgery to relieve their back pain even though such a major surgery would have little probability of allowing them to return to their stated goals of participation in a previously abandoned extreme sport, strenuous activity, or occupation. They automatically view surgery as an easier route than fully engaging in a rehabilitation program and modifying their activities in the meantime.

These patients don't play the odds. The likely outcome of surgery *will* be a modification of their activities, and if in fact they *did* modify their activities and added some proper rehabilitation, they would likely be able to avoid surgery and have the same outcome.

I certainly sympathize. As I mentioned earlier, my second knee surgery was prompted in large part by a desire to attain an idealized image of myself and my athletic abilities. I didn't realize that by appropriate training and some activity modification, I could attain a more than acceptable quality of life without surgery.

As a surgeon, this is one of the hardest discussions I have with patients. I try to understand where they are in their lives. This includes their ages, occupations, goals, and hobbies. After examining them and reviewing their diagnostic MRIs or X-rays, I try to weigh the risks and benefits of the different surgical tools at my disposal. I take into consideration my experience with the different surgical procedures and the cumulative outcomes of other patients with similar conditions on which I have operated. I try to predict the likely outcome, instead of being overly optimistic and seeing only the best-case surgical scenario.

As you can imagine, this is a very complicated calculus. It's not as if I know everything about the patient's life, and it's not as if they know everything I know about the surgery. The best decisions are made when we bridge this divide together. When the patient properly assesses their future life trajectory in light of their spine abnormality and options (surgical and non-operative), they often make the best long-term decision.

Similarly, since I have integrated non-operative treatment in my surgical practice, I am able to know more about the patient's characteristics and their goals. Therefore I am better able to guide patients in these difficult decisions. As a group, my team and I receive deeper engagement with these patients over multiple visits. I know that patients who have gone through the program have focused on maximizing function and not letting pain govern their lives. There is a concerted message, cautioning against catastrophizing and the lure of a quick fix. Importantly, patients have access to others with similar conditions who have learned to live with their circumstance without surgery, as well as those who are recovering from surgery.

In such a setting, it is easier for me to feel confident that the patient is making truly informed decisions about their care—that they realize how surgery will impact their ability to work or enjoy a hobby that they love. Are they willing to live happily without that hobby or work activity or are they willing to take a risk in order to keep pursuing it? Have they undergone the best non-operative treatment? Are they thinking correctly about their condition? These questions help the patient as well as their doctors figure out the proper approach to healing.

Challenge Your Tendency Toward Negative Thinking

From time to time, I still find that I am surprised by how completely a patient who I meet has become undone by the force of his fears and lack of good knowledge with which to make a decision about his care... and what an amazing and complete recovery he can accomplish when he masters them.

Several years ago, I met Jonathon, a 16-year-old tennis player who competed at state, regional, and national tournaments. He shared a coach with me and my kids. I watched him in action and hit with him on several occasions. The power and spin on his shots impressed me. Jonathon was all muscle.

So it seemed unusual when his dad contacted me six months later to tell me Jonathon was experiencing a great deal of back pain, so much so that he'd had to pull out of a recent tennis tournament. During my examination, he explained that it was his signature shots—his "kick serve" and his big backhand—that were giving him pain. Jonathon explained that he would have to bend quite a bit to generate the level of spin he needed on this serve and he had difficulty with the whip on his groundstrokes.

When I reviewed the MRI, his discs looked pretty good, but I did note some abnormalities in the facet joint, a small joint that works with the disc to provide motion in the spine. I gave him an injection in the facet, which seemed to provide some relief initially. However, a few months later, he had to pull out of another tournament due to pain. This was particularly distressing to him because he was working incredibly hard to raise his ranking to qualify for a tennis scholarship to Division I colleges. But despite a second injection, Jonathon's pain relief was only short-lived. Now was not the time to be missing tournaments and there were two more on the horizon. The pressure was on.

His father pressed for further intervention so that Jonathon wouldn't miss his moment. But I explained that surgery wasn't a good idea and further injections were likely not going to help. Jonathon was young and the anatomical abnormalities we'd identified in his back were not significant. So instead, I suggested that he skip the next tournament and instead spend the next four weeks balancing the strength of his trunk.

His father was skeptical. "Look at him!" he said. "He's in phenomenal condition. How could strengthening make a difference?" I explained to him that even though his son sported an admirable six pack, I was unconvinced his back muscles were strong and well-balanced enough to adequately support that power serve. The sidebar on the following page explains why.

BACK STRENGTHENING: A COMPLICATED CHALLENGE

The core muscles that support the back include the abdominal muscles in front as well as the obliques, which course along the side of the abdomen, but also very importantly, the muscles on the back itself. The back muscles include the superficial ones that are used for large motions (like Jonathon's tennis serve) to propel the trunk, but also the deep muscles that stabilize the vertebral bodies.

Building these stabilizing muscles is not easy. For example, in knee strain, the nervous system, in an attempt to prevent further injury to the knee joint, shuts down the quadriceps and even hip muscles. As a result, these stabilizing muscles quickly atrophy even after the strain improves, and it is very difficult to strengthen them again with regular daily activities and without specific exercises. This is the body's way of protecting against our inadvertent overuse of an injured body part and allowing us to heal.

Similarly, in cases of back pain, the deep muscles get selectively "turned off" and therefore are weaker than they should be. Unlike the quadriceps, which we can visibly assess and strengthen, the back muscles are much more complex and difficult to evaluate. This is why it is so important to have some type of objective test of strength for the back. It is important to know how strong those stabilizing muscles are compared to people of similar age, and to use such testing for continued assessment throughout rehabilitation to ensure a patient is making progress in strengthening.

In back pain, deep muscles get selectively "turned off" and are weaker than they should be.

So even though Jonathon had seen many physical therapists, chiropractors, and used a personal trainer, his father agreed that his back strength had never been measured. I also suspected that his catastrophizing and agitation about achieving his college dream was spilling over and contributing to his lack of progress. He was likely trying to muscle those serves over even more than he normally did, and his weak back was complaining. In trying to push through his pain, Jonathon was actually causing more trauma to his weakened spine.

If you're not aware of this imbalance in strength (as is true for most people), you can head into a downward spiral, where you experience greater pain and more inhibition of the back muscles, which then adds to your mental anguish in such situations. When we finally tested Jonathon's muscle strength on a computerized machine, we learned that despite his unbelievable strength in the rest of his body, he had below average strength in his back compared to other kids his age.

With strengthening that isolated those weaker muscles, he was able to bring his strength up to greater than one standard deviation above normal. (What does this mean exactly? It means that his strength was better than 70 percent of people. If he were two standard deviations above normal, his strength would be better than 98 percent of average people.)

As his strength approached this high to match the strength of the rest of his trunk, Jonathon quickly became pain free. Just three months later, he was able to shine at a critical national tournament and went on to receive a Division I scholarship at a great school. Thankfully he was willing to entertain the notion that, despite being in great physical condition, he could still be weak and imbalanced in certain muscles and therefore benefit from strengthening rather than seeking a drastic surgical option.

The Whole-Person Protocol: Seven Ways to Combat Negative Thoughts

When we talk about treating the "whole" person, it really begins with you and your ability to amass the best and most realistic scientific knowledge about your own body…and then bringing informed and tested methods as well as positive thoughts to bear on your recovery. It also involves facing your emotions and the role the mind plays in your physical well-being.

The good news is that you don't have to hire a cognitive behavioral therapist or have years of psychological treatment to become more aware of your negative thinking. Begin by searching for the truth instead of opinions; follow recommendations based on scientific proof when it is available. Most importantly, be sure to adopt a mindset of challenging negative thoughts and worries as they inevitably bubble up and see where that takes you. Here are a few methods for doing so:

Do a reality check. Pay particular attention to the recurrent thoughts you have as those likely have the most emotion attached to them. Face them, test them, dissect them, and most importantly, do so without added drama or emotion.

For example if you think, *I'm going to be debilitated by this condition. I probably won't work again,* you must dissect that thought. Is it really true? Take an inventory of what you can do. Are there really no jobs you can do if you worked your way up to it? How do you know? Have you tried everything in your power to allow for healing and better function, or are you letting the fear of pain dictate your efforts? What evidence do you see from observing others? Would your coworker or employer likely think the same thing? Would those who care for you want you to give up or fearfully rush into surgery?

By holding these thoughts up and examining them in the light of day, you bring fresh perspective to them.

In fact, ask friends and loved ones for their opinions. Take a quick poll of your most trusted confidants. Ask them how they see your situation and compare it with the thoughts you are having. Try not to focus on any one horror story or overly optimistic result and automatically assume that your outcome will be the same. Often, just by talking through your fears with other people, you can gain some perspective and get a handle on the truth.

Do your research. (Remember that knowledge is power.) Be assertive and engaged as you sift through the information that is shared about your condition and varied treatment protocols that are offered by different types of healthcare providers. Ask your chiropractor what lasting effect his treatment will have on your condition or your surgeon what will happen if you choose to forgo surgery. Seek others with a similar condition and expectations to ask how they did with their treatment.

Ask the experts your "worst-case scenario" questions. When you notice your mind heading to a worst-case scenario, ask directly, "Do you think I will continue to worsen and eventually be in a wheelchair due to this disc disease?" Then when a reliable source or sources (and don't be afraid to ask many different practitioners to get a consensus) responds, "Are you kidding? Of course not!" you can consciously let go of that concern.

Face your unpleasant feelings. If you are feeling angry or sad, ask yourself why you feel that way and sit with those feelings instead of pushing them away. Buried or unexpressed feelings have a way of manifesting in unexpected ways. I'm sure we have all experienced the transferring of emotion that can occur subconsciously. (For example, we try to suppress the feeling of annoyance when our spouse doesn't meet expectations for Valentine's Day, but we unwittingly take it out on them through undue criticism of another behavior.) By being honest with yourself and expressing your feelings, you will avoid overreacting in a sudden outburst to something unrelated or burying that emotion, which could then manifest in physical ailments.

Because our thoughts are often the source of our problems, forcefully trying to think differently can sometimes feel like fighting fire with fire. When you're feeling anxious, are catastrophizing, or your thoughts are racing, it will likely not work to just tell yourself to calm down. This is where meditation and gentle, loving understanding and observation without reaction can be so valuable to gain insight.

Seek tools that help to increase your awareness. When I have used the Vipassana insight meditation, I learned how to stop ignoring or avoiding my negative thoughts (which would just give them more power), in favor of allowing them to surface so I could observe them objectively. It took a significant investment of time and effort to obtain this very valuable tool, and to this day, I reap the benefits of learning how to meditate effectively. During this particular meditation, you first observe a physical sensation that comes welling up. It might be a pain or a pressure. Of course, it is attached to an emotion and a problem, but your goal is to focus only on the sensation itself.

By maintaining this present state of awareness, you will notice that the sensation and emotion both slowly dim. The beauty of this approach is that it is so simple and effective. You can address very complex issues by just focusing on the sensation. There are so many different centuries-old meditation traditions to choose from and many work very well. They range from mindfulness and guided visualization to Transcendental Meditation and simple focusing on your breath—so find what fits for you.

I believe that although it has clear benefits for some patients, in most cases there is no need to dissect issues from your childhood in psychotherapy to get relief from the anxiety associated with back pain. Anything that is disturbing you will naturally well up during the meditation. It can be uncomfortable at first as you observe it rising to the surface, but by the second or third time, you'll notice it has diminished. You will have essentially desensitized yourself to the difficult emotion, so it loses its power over you.

Allow healing to occur. Also, don't underestimate your body's ability to heal itself when appropriately treated. Cultivate patience by recognizing that years of neglect cannot be quickly reversed, but with patience, persistence, and appropriate stimulus, your body can compensate for many abnormalities. In fact, by participating in a mobilization/strengthening program, you can through your own experience demonstrate to yourself that your body is capable.

> *Your body can compensate for many abnormalities.*

I believe that things that bubble up in our lives—including physical ailments like back pain—are not a fluke. When they trigger strong feelings in us, it is likely because we have unresolved issues that need attention. They can worsen each time they arise in the form of similar events that threaten to overwhelm us. Pain in particular can frequently signal a sign of some imbalance we need to resolve and should be heeded as a wake-up call. Use this disturbance to improve your insight and life; it is there for a reason.

To continue our earlier gardener analogy from Chapter 2 (treat a sick patient the way a gardener treats an ailing plant), I encourage you to take a holistic approach to recovery when you have sustained a spinal injury or are suffering from chronic back or neck pain. Just as you would tend a plant with sun, oxygen, soil, and time to flourish, you must nourish the many facets of yourself to effect recovery. Feed your mind with accurate information and positive thinking. Then feed your body with exercise, periods of rest, and informed advice. Use intervention judiciously and with realistic expectations. In this way, you will truly harness your body's magnificent and innate ability to heal while also taking advantage of all of the great advances of modern medicine.

Key Learning Points: Treating the Whole Person

1. A proven treatment for chronic back pain includes recognizing the negative thoughts and feelings that occur when you have pain and learning how to change this negativity into healthy, positive thoughts and actions.
2. Seek out others with your similar condition and aspirations to ask about their experience with treatment, but be cautious in generalizing conditions or treatments that are dissimilar.
3. Don't underestimate your body's ability to heal itself when appropriately treated. Cultivate patience by recognizing that years of neglect cannot be quickly reversed, but with patience, persistence, and appropriate stimulus, your body can compensate for many abnormalities.

4. Seek scientific proof when it is available, value experience and proven treatments, and be wary of opinions and the latest fads in treatment.
5. Initiate a meditation practice to experience your thoughts and bodily sensations without reacting. Choose a style that fits best for you.

CHAPTER 5

UNDERSTANDING YOUR BACK AND DISPELLING MYTHS

> "Science is a way of thinking much more than it is a body of knowledge."
>
> —Carl Sagan

To take good care of our backs and ensure they serve us well into a pain-free old age, it's important to understand a little about them. I am about to get a bit "technical" in terms of how the back is constructed, how it moves, and why it is susceptible to certain injuries. Please bear with me. I truly believe that when you understand the "whys" behind a treatment regimen you'll be far more likely to adhere to it.

Later on I am also going to dispel some myths. However, I'll set the stage by addressing the biggest myth of all: that back pain is a normal part of aging. It's just not true.

It *is* true that, for better or for worse, we become susceptible to certain types of conditions as we age. For example, disc herniations become more and more common as we progress from 20 years old to about 45 years old. However, after that, discs generally collapse a bit as the result of the aging process. As the disc collapses and stiffens, there simply is less of it left to herniate. (For once, some good news for people over 45!)

The reality is that your back can serve you well into your golden years if you understand how to support good spinal health. I've seen many 80- and 90-year-old people who have worked and played often strenuously throughout their lives, but since they have taken care of their back, still enjoy golf and tennis.

To do that, you must understand how your spine is similar to other joints in your body and how it is different. So let's talk a bit about anatomy next, focusing only on important concepts that have practical implications for how to effectively rehabilitate the spine.

Your Spine: A Unique Set of Joints

For our purposes in understanding what works for rehabilitation, there are essentially four big differences between the joints of the back and the rest of the skeleton. These are:

1. **There are vital structures nearby and embedded within the structure of the spine.** The spinal cord and nerves pass between the discs in front and small joints (called the facet joints) in the back. This has an obvious implication. If you develop a growth such as a bone spur on your spine, it could easily pinch off nerves in the spinal canal and cause additional damage. This is clearly different than if

you had a bone spur on your knee, which might bulge out a bit, but it's not going to create a bigger problem by pinching another structure in the knee. Since the spinal cord and nerves are so close to the mobile discs, it's even more important to keep our discs healthy.

In the neck, a vital artery to the brain, called the vertebral artery, passes through a small tunnel in the bone. In elderly people, this artery can become compressed over time through degeneration that occurs with aging. Also, when plaque build-up occurs in these arteries, plaques can be dislodged with sudden movements. That's why it's very important during rehabilitation to avoid quick movements of the neck and to be aware of any symptoms that may occur during exercise or range of motion to avoid this as it can cause a stroke and severe neurological symptoms.

2. **The spine is like a chain with multiple joints.** The spine differs from other joints, like hip or shoulder joints, which are essentially comprised of one large ball and socket joint. In those joints, the two surfaces glide, one on top of the other, to provide a wide range of motion, while in the spine, multiple joints each move a little bit to provide range of motion. As a result, it is important that forces get distributed evenly and that no one joint get stressed too much.

There are some natural areas where stresses can accumulate, such as in the low back, and these stresses are amplified when our posture or lifting habits are poor. As a result of the increased force on these and adjacent spinal joints, you can experience early degeneration and increased pain.

As the body reacts to this increased force, it can lay down more soft tissue and bone, which can cause compression of traversing nerves (also called stenosis). Also, when one of the joints is stiff or welded together (fused surgically), it can create stress on adjacent spinal joints that can also degenerate more quickly.

Another implication of the spinal structure is that it is impossible to fully immobilize an injured area in the back in the way you could with a knee or ankle injury. This complex structure also makes it more difficult to isolate areas of weakness or specifically immobilize injured regions during rehabilitation.

The spine is like a chain with multiple joints.

3. **Discs are avascular.** In other words, except for a small outer portion, discs do not have a direct blood supply. This is in contrast to joints like the knee, for example, which have direct blood supply through the bone adjacent to the cartilage. In fact, the disc is the largest avascular structure in the whole body.

This has important implications for nutrition. Since there is no direct blood supply, nutrients diffuse in and waste products are pushed out of the disc partly by the pumping mechanism that occurs when we move. Hence it's important to feed the spine through movement, stretching, and exercise, or it will starve and degenerate sooner. Essentially, the more you move, the more adequately you infuse your spine with nutrients and help optimize its function.

This is why people of all ages—usually including those who are currently experiencing back pain—need to consciously make physical activity part of their life. I advise all patients to set a timer and get up briefly to stretch or take a short walk every half-hour. Additionally, getting adequate hydration (eight 8-ounce glasses of fluid a day) will also mean that you make more trips to the restroom—further ensuring that you get enough movement throughout your day.

One activity that I find especially helpful to maintain good spinal flexibility and health is a yoga-based exercise called "cat-cow." Do not perform this exercise if you have knee or wrist injuries, or are in acute severe back pain.

This exercise is done while kneeling on all fours with the knees directly under the hips and the wrists under the shoulders. Inhale and lengthen your spine, distributing the weight evenly to the hands and knees. Exhale and round your spine, pulling the abdominals in and tucking your pelvis under. This is the "cat" position. Next, inhale and rotate the tailbone toward the ceiling and the ribs and chest toward the floor. Lift your head and look to the ceiling. This is the "cow" position. Repeat these postures for five to ten breaths at least once a day.

4. **The spine is comprised of two sets of joints.** These are split up around the nerves, and what happens to one section causes a corresponding reaction in the other section, much like a seesaw,

where one side (the disc) rises as the other (the facet joint) falls. In the spine, as the disc is loaded, the facet joints are unloaded. When either of these gets stressed excessively, it can cause problems.

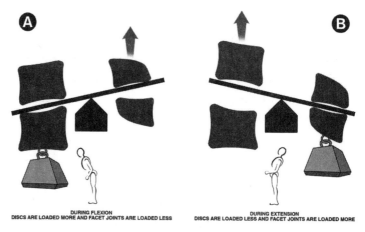

Image A: During flexion (bending forward), discs are loaded more and facet joints are loaded less. Image B: During extension (bending backward), discs are loaded less and facet joints are loaded more.

As a result, the front portion of the spine feels more pressure as you bend forward. (This is why repeated bending, prolonged slouching, or a sustained forward stoop strains discs for faster degeneration.) Bending backwards puts more pressure on the facet joints. If you are someone whose activity involves excessive extension—like our tennis player Jonathon or a gymnast—you can benefit from greater awareness of how the head aligns with the shoulders, hips, and knees as well as strengthening and

postural exercises to minimize strain on any one
area of the spine.

Bending backwards puts more pres-
sure on the facet joints.

How the Spine Is Similar to Other Joints

Throughout the many years I learned and then
taught about the spine, the differences between it and
other joints in the body were always emphasized. The
point was to understand that things we knew to be
true about other joints could not necessarily be applied
to the spine. And yet, the more I experienced and observed—both through consideration of my own knee
injuries and what I learned from treating patients in my
surgical practice and at SpineZone—the more I realized
there may be more similarities than differences.[1] This
suggests that the same type of treatments we know
work for the shoulder and the knee might also work
for the back—with some modifications to also take into
consideration the differences, of course.

For instance, a thin layer of cartilage covers the bone
in both the knee and the spine. Both joints also have a
capsule that surrounds them as well as ligaments and
hard structures that hold the joint together. And they
both have a mechanism that reduces friction with
movement, just as two ball bearings are lubricated by
oil when they move against each other.

The fluid-rich substance that separates discs in the
back is called the "nucleus" and is essentially 80 percent water. The nucleus is composed of a lattice that is

designed to suck up water, much like a sponge, to both lubricate and cushion any blow to the spine.

When you move against gravity as you walk or do other upright activities, you essentially push on this sponge, which squeezes a little bit of fluid outside of the disc. The water then gradually seeps back in when you release pressure on the joint during sleep, for example. This same process occurs with the fluid in your shoulder, knee, and other joints within the body that contain cartilage, but much less dramatically so.

This anatomic reality drives home a very important point about how much of our bodies are made of water and fluid, and how important adequate hydration is for function. Although I do not know of any studies that suggest that ingesting plenty of water would help disc hydration, it stands to reason that overall body hydration would be helpful for the discs of the spine.

WATER IS GREAT FOR HYDRATION. CAFFEINE AND ALCOHOL, NOT SO MUCH!

Hydration can be improved by sipping water throughout the day. Most of us realize how important it is to rehydrate after exercise or during particularly hot and dry days, of course, but we may not realize that we need to keep a big bottle of water on our desk and take a drink every 10 minutes or so. This is a habit everyone would do well to develop.

Reducing or eliminating the use of caffeinated drinks such as coffee and soda can also help, since these drinks actually contribute to dehydration. (I probably don't need to point out that there are many additional good reasons to cut down on these beverages—soda, in particular.)

Alcohol consumption should also be minimized. Not only does it decrease hydration, it is also a depressant and carries with it the potential for addiction. I have seen many patients who use alcohol to self-medicate. This starts a detrimental cycle of unhealthy food choices due to a booze-induced lack of self-control (as well as the empty calories of the alcoholic drink itself), decreased motivation to exercise, and even alterations in the quality of sleep.

There is plenty of evidence that the amount and type of load placed on any joint, including the disc, directly affects its hydration. Stooped posture has been shown to significantly decrease overall water content of the disc compared to erect postures.[2] Since the disc functions at its best when hydrated, posture has implications for injury mechanisms associated with stooped work, like gardening or even working at a desk with poor ergonomics.

Also, warming up prior to strenuous activity is important not only for the muscles, but for the anatomic characteristics of the disc. I was intrigued by a study on the loading of discs that makes perfect sense in regard to my patients. In this study, discs were noted to increase their shock absorptive capacity after 30 minutes of light load warm-up (a load equivalent to light manual labor), and the disc had a significant increase in its stiffness that plateaued after 30 minutes.[3] After two hours of continuous load equivalent to light manual labor, however, the disc was significantly less able to withstand stress and absorb shock.

Clinically this makes sense to me since many disc injuries often occur after either a quick or forceful motion before appropriate warm up, or after excessive sustained load. Even though this study was conducted in animals, it is very important to realize that your discs need to be primed by lighter activity and warm-up before moving on to more strenuous exertion. Also, it's very important to be careful to take breaks (and not continually load your discs for longer than two hours at a time) to let the discs rehydrate. These are common-sense lessons we have all heard before, but it is nice to know that there is an actual anatomic reason for it.

TIPS FOR IMPROVED DISC HEALTH DURING PHYSICAL ACTIVITY

1. It's vitally important to warm up prior to doing a strenuous activity. Pre-loading the disc at a lower resistance increases the ability of the disc to absorb stress and to avoid injury. For example, if you want to lift a heavy item,

lift a lighter item first so you can prepare the disc for a larger load.

2. Keep neutral posture as much as possible and avoid prolonged (greater than 15-20 minutes) stooped postures without breaks.

3. Realize that your disc hydration is highest at the beginning of the day and decreases steadily as gravity gradually squeezes more fluid out of the disc—so plan your activities accordingly and insert appropriate breaks for rehydration as the next points suggest.

4. Take frequent breaks (at least every hour) when sitting for long periods. The act of standing or stretching for even a few minutes allows fluid exchange in the disc.

5. Taking weight off of the spine, either through a full forward bend (which has the added benefit of stretching your hamstrings), pushing up on your arm rests, or lying down for two minutes every four hours will help rehydrate your discs. It is important to do this every two hours if you are doing continuous or repetitive bending and lifting. It's almost as if you are allowing that sponge, which is your disc, to reabsorb the fluid and swell. To back pain sufferers, a stiff spine feels more like a brittle dry bone, so it is important to restore that cushion to return the disc to the fluid-rich ecosystem it actually is.

> 6. If you are a long distance runner, you should take a break after every hour of running to rehydrate your discs. One study showed that discs undergo significant strain after one hour of running that, in the long term, may lead to low back pain and degenerative disc disease.[4]

As you can see, the disc is structured to use fluid and hydration to act as a shock absorber. Other joints in the body are also very well designed and engineered for the tasks they need to do. Each segment in the back has a remarkable built-in intelligence to assess the necessary trade-offs between mobility and stability.

Each segment in the back has a remarkable built-in intelligence to assess the necessary trade-offs between mobility and stability.

In the neck, for example, the top two vertebrae are responsible for 50 percent of all rotation, bending, and extension. To maintain this mobility, these segments rely on strong ligaments (not bony structures) to maintain stability. We rely upon vertebrae in the lower back for much of the motion when we bend; however the trade-off is that this puts increased strain on the ligaments and disc at this level.

This is similar to the shoulder, which is mobile in many directions, but its ligaments can loosen or tear, rendering it somewhat unstable. The bony structure of the shoulder contains a shallow socket to hold the ball of the arm bone. This allows for great range of motion, but requires the ligaments and muscles to be strong to keep the arm bone connected in its socket. In contrast, the hip bone contains a much deeper socket that cups around the ball of the hip joint, keeping it stable.

Just as it's easier to tear tendons in a shoulder because of this inherent instability, so it is also easy to injure certain areas of the back that are the focus of more motion. This is why people develop and are more prone to develop slippage of the vertebrae or spondylolisthesis, a spine problem we discussed earlier, at L4-5 where the stress is concentrated. The concentrated motion and increased stress loosen the disc and ligaments and result in the development of instability and slippage in the lower spine. Similarly, since more force and motion is concentrated there, the C5-6 is the most common disc to degenerate first.

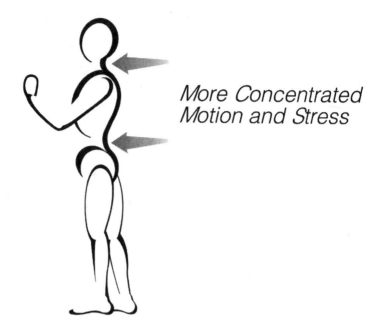

*More Concentrated
Motion and Stress*

The neck and low back provide a lot of motion, but their linkage to large areas—such as the head, chest, and pelvis—causes stress to accumulate in them.

How Muscles Stabilize Your Frame

Each joint in your body has muscles that are uniquely designed to stabilize it and are quick to atrophy when there's an injury to them. In the knee, it's the "vastus medialis oblique," or VMO, part of the quadriceps muscle, as well as the gluteus medius (a hip muscle), which stabilizes and helps align the kneecap and knee in general. The VMO is known to atrophy quickly with an injury, and patients with weak gluteus medius and VMO muscles are known to develop knee instability.

Each joint in your body has muscles that are uniquely designed to stabilize it and are quick to atrophy when there's an injury.

In the shoulder, it's the rotator cuff strength that is pivotal to shoulder stability, without which early shoulder arthritis and ligament tearing will develop. And in the back, it's a muscle called the "multifidus." These muscles are each essential to shielding the respective joints from stress by actively stabilizing them during motion. They are the common denominator for preventing injury through strengthening because they are stabilizers.

It is well established that the VMO is important in ensuring the kneecap tracks correctly. In healthy individuals, this short and stout muscle is active throughout the range of motion. It fires first to stabilize the patella, followed by the other quadriceps and hip muscles, which power the motion. But when there is knee dysfunction and pain, it fires late and inconsistently.

However, in patients with knee pain, the VMO fatigues easily and is quick to atrophy (i.e., shrink in size and strength). Similarly, the gluteus medius muscle of the hip stabilizes the thigh bone so it does not rotate out of alignment and put more stress on the knee. Strengthening of these muscles is a key part of rehabilitating knee injuries. As the muscles regain their strength, the pain in the knee often subsides.

Similar to the gluteus medius and VMO is the multifidus in the back. It is a small, stout muscle that stabilizes the vertebrae while other muscles move the trunk. One study showed that, in comparison with healthy subjects, chronic low back pain patients displayed significantly lower activity of the multifidus muscle during coordination exercises.[5] The authors concluded that multifidus dysfunction may be at least partly to blame for the onset of pain, its recurrence, or continued pain.[6] We will discuss the role of this important multifidus muscle in more detail later in this chapter.

When these key stabilizing muscles around the joints are stronger, the joints are better able to tolerate stresses. This is why it's important to have a general understanding of functional anatomy. While your body is very well designed to serve you, it's important to be aware of the load you are placing on less stable parts of your spine. Over time, shoulders, knees, and the spine are prone to injury. As such, it's important to be proactive about protecting these joints so they remain strong and pain-free in old age.

Along with many of my orthopedic colleagues, I recommend that anyone over 40 make strengthening the stabilizing muscles of the shoulder and the knee a priority to avoid injury for this very reason. The American Academy of Orthopaedic Surgeons offers some great information on strengthening these essential muscle groups. To access them, check out www.orthoinfo.org.

In the same way, back strengthening—particularly targeting the multifidus—will help you avoid the cascade of degeneration that so commonly causes an unstable spine later in life. (We'll discuss back strengthening further in Chapter 6.)

Other Important Anatomic Factors

The "shock absorbers" of the joints—the cartilage in knees or the discs of the spine, for example—are anatomically built to withstand gravity's forces. But there is an important caveat: When directly loaded, such as when we walk or run, both the spinal disc and the knee cartilage can withstand many times your body weight.

However, if the spine load is coming at an angle, such as when you carry something with arms outstretched, far from your body, or in the knee, when you try to change directions suddenly, the disc and cartilage are at much more risk and less able to withstand the forces.[7]

Another big factor that changes the load and distribution of stress to the spine is body weight. Since men carry their weight up front in their middle section, having a large stomach applies an uneven forward pull to the spine. This causes more strain on the back muscles and discs. Similarly, women with large breasts have increased strain on their upper back and neck muscles and discs.

This is also a good time to talk about maintaining a normal body weight. Obesity is an important factor in developing disc disease. Body mass index (BMI) over 25 is strongly associated with increased risk of disc degeneration.[8] Importantly, being overweight from a younger age is an even stronger predictor of premature disc degeneration.

If you are overweight, know that you are likely to experience or continue experiencing back pain further down the road. I urge you to make every effort to lighten this excess strain on your discs now, so you don't have regrets later. I absolutely cannot stress this point strongly enough. While a thorough discussion of weight loss is beyond the scope of this book, we will cover a few helpful tips for achieving and maintaining a healthy body weight in the "best practices" chapter at the end of this book.

Another structural issue to understand is that, at birth, about 80 percent of the disc is water. Then, as we age, these discs begin to dehydrate and become less supple. However, the good news is that as we age, the inflammatory proteins in the disc also diminish. As a result, discs typically become less painful after age 60. Why is this important? Because it's one more reason to consider waiting out a disc problem. As you age, it will likely become less painful as it naturally becomes stiffer. When we fuse a disc in surgery, we are essentially accelerating a natural process that would occur over time.

> *Discs typically become less painful after age 60.*

Feeding Your Spine

As we have seen, the disc is the largest avascular structure in the body (i.e., lacking direct blood supply). However, in children, it is actually well vascularized. As a result, kids' discs heal much more quickly from injuries. In adults, however, there is blood supply only to the outer 1-2 millimeters of the disc; the remaining nutrients must find other ways into the disc.[9]

In adults, for discs to receive nutrition, oxygen and glucose flowing in the blood must make their way to the edges of the vertebrae next to the disc. From there, the oxygen and glucose must seep through small capillaries inside the endplates of the vertebrae into the nucleus. In a healthy spine, large molecules like growth factors, proteins, and breakdown products can't just seep in; instead, they are pushed in and pulled out of the disc through motion in a continual process of pumping in nourishment and pumping out waste.

This inflow and outflow is so remarkable that the disc height actually gets as much as 25 percent shorter at the end of each day as the pressure of gravity compresses the discs in the spine. (You can demonstrate this to yourself by checking your height in the morning and comparing it at the end of the day. Height can decrease as much as three-quarters of an inch daily. Astronauts actually gain a few inches in height due to the absence of gravity. Their discs swell.)

Smoking and vibration (i.e., from driving) also diminish blood flow; they cause the small blood vessels at the ends of the vertebral bodies to become constricted so that they cannot diffuse blood nutrients to the spine. When this occurs, disc injuries and degeneration can result from the starving of the disc cells and hardening of the adjacent bone, which can further hamper nutrition to the disc. (Another good reason not to smoke—as if you needed one more!)

Likewise, the blood supply to the edges of the vertebrae decreases as you age. To see how critical the blood supply is to good spinal health, we need only look to elderly patients with atherosclerosis of the aorta. In such cases, the arteries that extend from the aorta to the spine are thickened from plaque build-up. Due to the decreased blood supply, these patients quickly develop progressive disc degeneration.

The lesson is clear. If you want to keep your spine healthy, do everything possible to slow the aging process: stop smoking, eat healthful foods (to combat atherosclerosis), and get plenty of exercise. You can't entirely stop the ravages of Father Time, of course, but you can do a lot to delay them and keep them to a minimum.

Now that you have a basic understanding of the functional anatomy of the spine, what nourishes it, and what causes problems, let's examine several myths about back pain and how they relate to the structure of your back.

Myth #1: "Bed rest is necessary when someone is in severe back pain."

A concern I hear patients commonly express is that if they have severe back pain, they must need to rest it until the pain abates. In their minds, severe pain must equate to severe structural damage, which is not true. As we reviewed earlier, there are many factors that create an individual's perception of pain. So just because someone is experiencing a lot of pain, they do not necessarily have a severe or serious injury or spinal defect.

Resting the back in bed to reduce pain is a myth we need to bust. Beyond a few days after an injury, bed rest is not helpful. It may even worsen the long-term deconditioning of the spine because you'll need to work that much harder to restore muscle that atrophied due to the extra days in bed. Individuals who are convinced they need bed rest can often become fearful about moving and depressed as they begin to catastrophize about what is causing the pain and imagine worst-case scenarios.

> *Resting the back in bed to reduce pain*
> *is a myth.*

In fact, back pain patients can significantly benefit from aggressive rehabilitation, which goes well beyond physical therapy, but yet is monitored by a physician and performed in a controlled manner not to worsen the underlying condition. As reported in the *Wall Street Journal*, patients who can commit themselves to this process are far more likely to return to work, have less pain, and are less likely to seek additional back treatment.[10] A day or two to calm pain is acceptable, but after that it's important to slowly resume activity, which brings us to another myth...

Myth #2: "Lifting and exercise cause back pain."

In addition to resting in bed, many people think they should also avoid lifting anything if they have a bad back, but this too is a myth. Your back muscles will grow weaker if you don't use them, as I noted. Just ensure you lift correctly so you are strengthening instead of straining when you use them.

In the same way, exercising incorrectly *can* cause back pain and disc injuries. This is common in people who use high-intensity, short-duration workouts. As they begin to fatigue, their posture falters...they may unconsciously lift with their back in a flexed position instead of using their strong hip muscles, for example. For this very reason, I now see an unusual increase in otherwise very fit 25- to 35-year-old patients with back pain and disc herniations. (An important rule of thumb: If you can't do a repetition with perfect posture, don't do it!)

If you are a weekend warrior—meaning you train hard only a few consecutive days a week and are otherwise generally sedentary—you can injure your spine and most other joints if you are not careful. Remember how I injured my knee by pushing too hard without proper conditioning during my college days? Your workouts should be spaced throughout the week on a suitable schedule. It is also important to work your way up in terms of intensity, because we aren't meant to go from 0 to 60 after days of inactivity. Further, in order to keep your back muscles strong and conditioned, your spine actually needs regular stretching and strengthening.

In fact, studies show that long-term exercise (greater than three months) has a significant impact on disc health due to a significantly higher rate of sulfate and oxygen transport into the disc, likely by improving the microcirculation of the ends of the vertebral body that feed the disc.[11] In short, exercise not only primes the pump by directly driving nutrients into the disc, but also by filling the pipes through increased blood flow that carries those nutrients to the disc.

This is why exercise is all the more critical for patients with spine disorders and deformities. In scoliosis, for example, the apex—the point of the most curvature in the spine—receives the least nutrition. Exercise is an important way to combat the natural progression of such disorders and slow the rate of further degeneration.

Myth #3: "Repetitive bending causes back pain."

It's true that if you consistently don't bend *correctly*, you can cause accelerated degeneration of discs in both the lower and upper sections of your spine. However, there is a common misconception that individuals who do a lot of repetitive bending each day will *always* develop an injury.

In fact, many individuals in China, Africa, and rural farming areas that bend many times daily still maintain exceptionally healthy backs. This is because they bend through their hips, rather than through their backs. Your hips are built with a more stable joint and a wider range of motion for just such a movement. By keeping your back flat with a slight lordosis (normal curve) and "hinging" at your hip as you bend, you can protect your lower spine. It's all about bending correctly.

**PROPER BENDING
LIFTING**

**IMPROPER BENDING
LIFTING**

It's important to maintain lumbar lordosis and pelvic anteversion (in the left-hand graphic above, the arrow depicts the proper counterclockwise rotation of pelvis) when bending or lifting. Even if you bend forward, as long as you bend thru the hips and maintain at least a flat spine or slight lumbar lordosis, this protects the back. Note that you will need to have limber hamstrings to be able to bend this way. Alternatively, you can squat when bending or lifting; however, be careful to continue to maintain the lumbar lordosis and not try to lift too much on one side (i.e., it's best to lift equal amounts in both hand to balance the forces on the spine). If you allow the "C" curve to develop while bending (whether squatting or not), it markedly increases the stress on your spine.

Bending incorrectly does indeed carry consequences. In fact, one of the emerging epidemics in spinal health is "text neck." The human head weighs about 12 pounds, which doesn't sound like much, until you bend forward and increase the weight on your neck. In a recent study, Dr. Ken Hansraj, chief of spine surgery at New York Spine Surgery and Rehabilitation Medicine, explains that when you tip your head 15 degrees, that 12 pounds feels like the equivalent of 27 pounds to your neck joints and muscles.[12] At 30 degrees, it's 40 pounds, and at 60 degrees it's 60 pounds. Sixty pounds is the equivalent of carrying an 8-year-old around your neck for a few hours every day.[13]

One of the emerging epidemics in spinal health is "text neck."

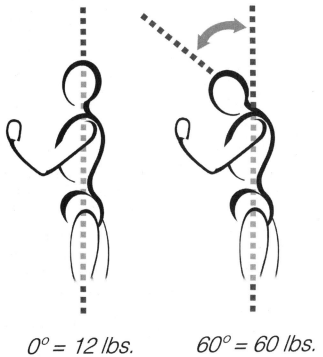

$0° = 12$ *lbs.* $60° = 60$ *lbs.*

The weight of the head is 12 lbs. as long as proper posture is maintained. When bending forward, the weight of the head can be as high as 60 lbs.

When your posture is suboptimal, your muscles have to work overtime—even though you may not realize it is happening at the time. Imagine balancing a broomstick upside down. You can actually balance it in the palm of your hand if you make fine adjustments to keep the stick vertical. That's essentially what your pelvis does to balance your head, neck, shoulders, and body. But if you were to try to hold that broomstick at a 45-degree angle, you'd need to grip it pretty hard because of the way the weight would be distributed. In the same way, over time, your back will have to work that much harder as it tries to hold its position with poor posture.

How far do *you* bend your neck when you text? According to research by Dr. Hansraj, billions of us are spending two to four hours a day in this position sending texts or reading email on our mobile devices, which will lead to excessive wear and tear on the spine, including muscle strain, pinched nerves, herniated discs, and more.[14] This is a perfect example of a seemingly insignificant repetitive motion that yields lasting negative results. So next time you pick up your smartphone, hold it higher, look down with your eyes, and avoid bending your neck!

Myth #4: "Pain is caused by joints being 'out of place.'"

Sometimes patients are under the impression that some joint must have "popped out"...that some type of misalignment (or subluxation) is the cause of lower back pain. However, there is no evidence that there are true subluxations of the joints in the back when there is pain. In addition, there is little evidence that disc bulges are related to lower back pain. (In fact, the vast majority of people have disc bulges with little to no pain.)

Yet, it's true that some patients report relief from spinal manipulations by chiropractors.

There is little evidence that disc bulges
are related to lower back pain.

I value chiropractic treatment and routinely refer both acute and selected chronic pain patients to chiropractic care for episodes of short-term care. These quick (high-velocity) and short (low-amplitude) manipulations can accelerate the improvement of range of motion in cases where joints are stiff.

However, I do not believe we need long-term, sustained, maintenance-based chiropractic manipulation for a healthy spine. (Our bodies have adapted over thousands of years of evolution to meet our wide range of needs for movement. No animal has ever needed chronic chiropractic care to maintain spinal health, so why would humans?)

It's likely that in the case where individuals report the benefits of chiropractic care that they are actually getting relief through the restoration of normal joint and muscle movements (rather than popping something back into place). When a chiropractor pops a joint in your back, it releases endorphins to produce a temporary "feel good" sensation, just as it does when you pop a knuckle in your hand. I find, however, that the passive process of manipulation does not result in longstanding improvement unless it is accompanied by postural awareness and strengthening.

Myth #5: "Scans are necessary to know exactly what the problem is."

In earlier chapters, you read about a number of patients who were a little obsessed with what their X-ray or MRI scans showed, even though the defects captured on those scans were not necessarily indicative of the problem. Remember Steve from Chapter 4? He was concerned about a disc herniation on an MRI scan that turned out to have nothing at all to do with the weakness in his foot.

His problem was due to diminished nerve function crossing at his knee. While it may seem intuitive that scans would provide clear evidence of pain, this is not frequently the case. The body is complex. The spine is complex. Our perceptions of pain are complex. So it's just not that clear cut.

The truth is that we can't always rely only on what we see on an MRI or X-ray to determine whether structural defects—or other factors—are truly causing the problem. Rather, imaging offers clues to consider in our diagnosis, and we must correlate the findings with the patient's symptoms.

In scoliosis, for example, many individuals have curvature of the spine with absolutely no symptoms and full function. (In fact, James Blake, a professional tennis player, was ranked number four in the world in singles at the height of his career despite a diagnosis of severe scoliosis when he was 13 years old. He wore a back brace in those days for 18 hours a day, except for when he was playing tennis. He had no pain.)

In addition to spondylolisthesis and scoliosis, disc herniations also fit this model. Using a jelly-filled donut analogy for the disc, when a disc herniates, it's as if the inner jelly portion has popped out onto a nerve. On an MRI scan, the nerve can look severely compressed. And yet, many individuals with large disc herniations on the MRI have no symptoms of pain while others with mild herniations are in so much pain they require surgery.

Even individuals who have never had pain in their lives will often show evidence on an MRI of degeneration and herniations. In fact, in a study of MRIs in people with an average of 42 years of age without back pain, only 36 percent had normal discs at all levels.[15] Clinical judgment when interpreting an MRI scan is paramount.

So, a structural problem on an MRI does not always indicate the presence of symptoms or need for surgery. Even in those patients who are experiencing significant pain and have abnormal MRI findings, non-operative treatment can transform them into asymptomatic patients with abnormal MRI findings. That's because individuals are unique and bring many genetic, environmental, and other factors to a problem that must be considered holistically.

> *A structural problem on an MRI does not always indicate the presence of symptoms or need for surgery.*

And yet, patients still assume that if the MRI shows evidence that something is wrong, then the MRI must be right and the abnormality must be fixed. This perception is perhaps not surprising because it's true that when an X-ray illuminates a fracture, we can better determine if the patient either needs a cast or surgery. When a lab test identifies heart muscle damage or an angiogram shows a tight coronary artery, we know we must address it. However, this is just not true when it comes to an MRI of the spine.

In most cases of lower back pain, X-rays are also unnecessary. Another important factor to consider: X-rays and CT scans expose patients to significant radiation. For instance, in a given year, all of us receive about 300 mrem (a unit used to measure the effect of radiation on the human body) of exposure to background radiation. A lumbar 4-view X-ray provides 300 mrem (essentially adding another background year of radiation) and a CT scan of the spine provides an additional 1,000 mrem. These extra studies can also lead to unnecessary treatment when an abnormality that does not actually pose a threat is identified on a scan. (Just think back to Nancy's story from Chapter 4. She ended up with multiple surgeries for a herniated disc found on an MRI that would have likely resolved on its own.)

Fortunately, a thorough clinical examination by a trained practitioner is usually the best way to identify those few patients who should have scans. The fact is that scans are usually meaningless when considered in isolation, for all the reasons you have read about thus far.

Because so many of us are eager to grasp onto an anatomical anomaly to explain and legitimize our pain, it's critical that health professionals use care and caution in how they talk about the results of such scans to patients. When we don't do a good job of this (and too often we don't), our patients may experience unnecessary fear, stress, and anxiety. And, as we have seen, our emotions play such a huge role in our actual clinical outcomes. So it's important to remain rational and realistic about the causes of pain. Otherwise, you will fall prey to the next myth:

Myth #6: "Back pain means that I will eventually need surgery."

Most people will experience back pain at some point during their lifetime, and 10 percent of the population will suffer chronic back pain—yet less than 1 percent of those chronic back pain patients will undergo surgery. This means according to even the relatively aggressive U.S. standard (which is double the rate in Canada, Western Europe, and Australia, and five times the rate in the United Kingdom[16]), only 1 in 1,000 people require surgery.[17] The vast majority of patients improve with no treatment or more conservative treatments like anti-inflammatory medications, exercises, coping skills, and strengthening.

How do you know if you may need surgery? Indications include nerve impingement that results in progressive weakness and tumors or infection. Also, patients with "refractory pain"—chronic pain that persists despite all attempts to treat it—can in certain circumstances benefit from surgery. But to be identified as such, the patient must have exhausted all other options, including a comprehensive, measurement-based, and targeted strengthening, stretching, and postural awareness program.

Myth #7:"Surgery will cure my back pain."

It's understandable that when we are in pain, we'd like to believe there is a quick and definitive solution to fixing it. Sometimes patients are sure that solution is surgery, even when it is not clinically indicated. Spine surgery is very effective in some cases (e.g., correcting deformities, treating instability, curing infections, stabilizing fractures, treating some tumors, and removing compression from nerves).

For example, in cases where a nerve is severely compressed and is causing arm or leg pain—and all non-operative treatment has failed—surgery can often cure the extremity pain. When the source of back pain is unclear, however, outcomes from spine surgery are not consistently better than outcomes from more conservative interventions.[18]

In other words, without a clear reason for the pain such as instability, nerve compression, or a fracture, surgery to treat a bad-looking disc on an MRI has a bad track record. A large proportion of patients experience only partial relief or even report that their pain is worse after surgery for back pain when it is performed for only a "dark" or dried-out disc on the MRI.

> *Without a clear reason for the pain, surgery to treat a bad-looking disc on an MRI has a bad track record.*

Operating on patients with dark discs and "non-descript" back or neck pain is becoming an increasingly common practice in the industry today. But these surgeries—though simple to justify—are often unsuccessful at ultimately relieving pain. Curtailing this increasingly accepted surgical practice is the "lowest hanging fruit" in terms of fixing our collective treatment of spinal conditions. For those times when there is no overwhelmingly clear indication for surgery (which is the vast majority of cases), we need a systematic approach or protocol for non-operative treatment that is able to reduce the occurrence of these less effective surgeries.

Like many other spine surgeons, I too have had some excellent, memorable results when treating patients with back pain caused by an isolated disc abnormality with fusion or disc replacement surgery. However, when objectively looking at the results, it becomes clear that this population has a much lower success rate than others. Some spine surgeons refuse to operate on patients with only neck or back pain. In my opinion, *some* of these patients would truly benefit from surgery, but only a minority—a well-selected subgroup of them.

It's important to examine the risks and benefits before choosing surgery. Just as we saw in the case of Nancy in Chapter 4, it makes so much more sense to see what the natural outcome of a condition is…that is, what would happen if we were to let the body cure itself without surgical intervention. Even better, what would happen if we maximized the body's ability to cure itself? In Nancy's case, the disc herniation causing her arm pain was resolving; however, she did not wait to maximize the natural outcome.

Once your body has reached its maximum potential for recovery on its own, see if you still feel that your current level of function is unacceptable. Only then should you compare the risks of surgery to the downsides of remaining in your current state. In many adult deformities, which often start in adolescence and progress with age, this calculus is even more complicated since the risks of this type of surgery are often very high.

In these cases, the risk of surgery needs to be weighed against how functional a patient can become with a comprehensive strengthening and stretching program, since not all therapy is equally effective in maximizing the body's coping mechanisms. Unless you have a serious problem with instability or nerve impingement where you are likely to worsen without surgery, choose the option for rehabilitation first. The potential for resolving your pain is excellent.

Myth #8: "Once I injure my back, full recovery is not possible."

One of the biggest fears I see in many of my patients is that they are destined to suffer back pain for the rest of their lives, based on a particularly painful neck or back injury. Actually, though, most people recover quite quickly, with a great deal of improvement occurring over the first few weeks post-injury and the rest resolving over the next few months.

Take comfort from the fact that most people who get back pain can experience it as a short-lived phenomenon and quickly return to work, hobbies, and other daily activities fully and without long-term restriction. There is a small minority of people who *will* develop chronic pain, but by addressing your condition early and appropriately, you can avoid being one of them. Of course, if you are concerned about your pain and exhibit "danger signs" like fever, chills, unexplained weight loss, or night pain, get evaluated by a physician, as these symptoms could indicate something more serious such as an infection or even cancer.

In Summary

Hopefully by now you are beginning to get a sense of the real reasons that you and others experience back pain, based on a better understanding of how the back works as a complex joint and what it needs from you to remain healthy: strength, stability, and movement. Good posture and appropriate exercise are key ingredients in helping your back help you.

When you add this understanding of your anatomy to what we learned in Chapter 2 about the many other unique psychological and physiological factors that contribute to an individual's perception of pain, you can begin to see why a specialized approach to treating back pain is so important.

If any of the preceding myths resonated for you, now is the time to set them aside so you can start to focus on exactly how to move forward with an effective and realistic plan to optimize strengthening. That's where we're headed next.

Key Learning Points: Understanding Your Back and Dispelling Myths

1. Your spine is unique from other joints in many ways: Vital structures such as nerves and arteries are embedded in the structure of the spine. The disc does not have good blood supply. There are areas of stress concentration that are more prone to instability if we are not careful.

2. Like other joints, the spine has stabilizing muscles—most notably, the multifidus—that protect it from injury. Keeping this muscle strong is important for back health.

3. For spinal discs to receive nutrition, there must be a healthy exchange of nutrients and waste products. Smoking, vibration (e.g., from driving), and bad posture all compromise this process; mobility and exercise enhance it.

4. There are abundant "myths" that circulate about back pain. These include: extended rest is necessary to treat back pain; repetitive bending causes back pain; pain is caused by joints being "out of place"; lifting and exercise cause back pain; scans are always necessary to uncover the problem; back pain means you'll eventually need surgery; surgery will cure back pain; and once you injure your back, full recovery is impossible. None of these are true!

5. While strengthening other joints is relatively straightforward, so-called "core" and home exercises frequently fall short in isolating the particular stabilizing muscles in the back.

6. When you *do* exercise, it's critical to use correct posture to avoid straining the wrong muscles.

MOVE BEYOND BACK PAIN

I n the previous chapters, we talked about the factors that make each of us physically unique, including the complex nature of how we perceive pain and the strong connection between the mind and body. In the same light, we discussed how important it is to consider the whole person when making treatment decisions and how our physical anatomy and emotional life both contribute to the challenges we experience.

With this as our foundation, let's turn our attention now to the practical tips we can use to take back control, to move beyond back pain. (Actually, we have covered some of these "how-tos" already, and Section 2 will provide even more of them. In fact, Chapter 9 will pull together many of the practical tips that have been provided throughout the book and put them in context for you to start using right now.)

What works to heal back or neck pain? In the past 20 years, I have seen many fads gain popularity, only to then fade into obscurity. There is ever-changing "noise" coming from surgeons, physical therapists, chiropractors, and more...essentially, from every one of the different disciplines that treat the back. It is amazing to me how many of these treatments, which initially appeared to be very promising, did not ultimately withstand the practical testing of others and the force of scientific scrutiny.

As someone with extensive training and experience surgically treating patients with advanced spinal conditions, I have been amazed how patients with these seemingly different conditions (and ones that I was taught would typically require surgery) have been able to avoid surgery or injections with simple restoration of spinal core muscle strength.

Of course, there is no single method that will work for all spine patients or for all conditions. However, it is still important to stick to key principles—such as improving strength and flexibility and maintaining good alignment and posture—even if it feels elusive or initially impossible to patients who are struggling with a lot of pain. That's why my SpineZone team and I have spent the past decade developing, honing, and field-testing exercises that help patients meet these goals.

We have seen many success stories over the years, and I am convinced that you can be one of them. Focusing on core spinal strengthening and flexibility can begin to untie all of the knots that back pain has caused in your life. By experiencing your spine's improvement in function and strength, you will focus less on pain and any negative thoughts about your spinal condition or MRI findings.

This book will provide some simple exercises, techniques, and good-habit-building practices you can try at home. Of course, it's not always as easy as it sounds to isolate the spinal core muscles and to strengthen them efficiently. Flexibility and postural balance are important factors to consider as well. If you find going it alone doesn't work for you, I hope you will seek out a multi-specialty clinic that not only teaches you the right exercises but also educates you and provides psychological and social support.

Our healthcare system is replete with excellent practitioners in their individual fields, yet not always working in a coordinated fashion. The good news is that this model is quickly changing, as it should. An integrated approach to spine care (one that employs reproducible, measurable methods that can be tested and verified for efficacy, patient satisfaction, and cost) is very much aligned with the transformation the healthcare industry is currently undergoing.

With all of this in mind, let's talk next about spine strengthening as our best option to relieve pain long-term: what you need to know and how to optimize an integrated plan for success. I hope the information and advice in the pages ahead provide some relief from your pain and will result in a stronger, healthier, and happier you.

CHAPTER 6

GETTING STRONGER AND STRAIGHTER

"Out of difficulties grow miracles."

—Jean de La Bruyère

In this chapter, we talk about different components of spinal function and health. We will cover how the muscles of the back support the spine and explore the systems that work together to keep your back strong and healthy. We will also discuss the value of strengthening the spine and the ways that people may be unknowingly doing themselves harm.

Alex's Story: Superstar Athlete Hobbled by Suboptimal Back Strength

A number of years ago, I had the pleasure of reconnecting with an inspiring former patient of mine: Alex, a 23-year-old professional tennis player who was experiencing a lot of back and leg pain. I'd first met Alex several years prior when he was in college at a high-level Division I school. With his senior year of college tennis approaching, he wanted a solution to his persistent back and radiating buttock pain. At that time, his MRI had revealed a disc herniation, and therefore he underwent a discectomy surgery after injections had not been helpful.

After the discectomy surgery, his back and leg pain improved significantly, and he was able to return to playing in international competitions. In fact, he turned out some impressive performances in the pros. But then, just as his career was taking off, he had to drop out of one Grand Slam tournament due to significant back and radiating pain again.

That's when he consulted me a second time. But after reviewing new MRI scans, I told Alex that it was unlikely any new disc herniation was the culprit. I explained that he likely needed to adjust his conditioning regimen, which surprised him since he had the best of the best when it came to training through the U.S. Tennis Association (USTA) as well as a cadre of personal training coaches.

He was under a very strict exercise regimen, which included many core exercises and a personalized fitness plan. Before recommending continued treatment, I even visited the USTA training facility in Florida and spoke with his trainer to better understand where the problems might lie. It was clear to me, though, that his back muscles were out of balance.

So here in San Diego, we took him through a program where we isolated and measured the strength of his back muscles. Interestingly, we found his back muscles to be much weaker than expected. In fact, even with all of his conditioning and personal training as a professional tennis player, Alex had strength comparable to the lowest 2 percent of men his age without back pain! How could this be?

While he had a world-class forehand and could generate a power-packed serve over 110 miles per hour, the critical smaller stabilizing muscles were not doing their job stabilizing the spine. The good news is that with appropriate strength training that focused on the right muscles, we were able to quickly improve Alex's strength until he was up to the 20th percentile of normal in six weeks. Within three months of strengthening, his back strength returned to a level similar to the average normal population for his age.

And, as his measurable strength improved, so did his corresponding function and results on tour. Alex is an excellent example of just how critical core strengthening can be and also how difficult it can be to obtain the right kind of strengthening when there is underlying pain that is inhibiting normal function and the balance of muscles.

Tennis—like golf—is a very asymmetric sport, so it can put uneven strain on the back. Core muscle strength in such sports, as with any physical activity, is so important to proper functioning and prevention of injury. Once back pain does occur, though, it can be challenging even for a professional like Alex to appropriately isolate and improve the function of these deep back muscles.

Of course, you don't have to be a professional athlete for this asymmetry and weakness to affect you. Have you ever considered the cumulative toll that years of carrying a serving tray takes on a server's spine? Or how about the damage done when a student always carries a backpack on the same shoulder? Even rotating your neck in the same direction at your desk each day carries lasting consequences. Examples like these show how weakened stabilizing muscles contribute greatly to the development of chronic back pain in the general population. That's why the right approach—one that diagnoses and corrects deficits in stability, center of gravity, and muscle imbalances—is so critical, as we shall see.

Why do athletes like Alex, who are in great physical condition and have access to the best trainers and therapists, develop back and neck pain? Why are core muscle weakness and back pain so prevalent in these conditioned athletes? And for that matter, why are they so prevalent in the general population? With easily accessible exercises like sit-ups or floor exercises—or even manual assistance to strengthen the core—why can't these patients suffering from back pain manage to build up the appropriate amount of strength to support their spines?

There are four main reasons most people have not developed an optimal amount of back strength: 1) the main stabilizing muscles of the spine become weakened with age—particularly in patients with chronic pain who voluntarily or involuntarily shut down their back muscles, 2) with standard core exercises it is difficult to control the resistance through the entire range of motion and to sequentially apply a measurable, heavier resistance, 3) many people lead sedentary lifestyles and/ or have spine-weakening bad posture, both of which can lead to permanent problems, and 4) it takes hard work to build muscle.

Now, let's dig a little deeper to get to the core of these four issues:

1. **Both age and injury prevent the strengthening of key stabilizing muscles.**

   There is a very significant difference that needs to be taken into account when strengthening the core spinal muscles versus other muscles in the body. The core muscular system is divided into two components: a local system with deep, stout muscles that run between each vertebrae and act to stabilize them, and a system with longer muscles that span many different vertebrae, allowing them to propel the spine and generate motion of the entire body.

   In several studies, authors used computer and physical models of the cervical spine to show that activating only large, long muscles resulted in instability, especially with respect to upright posture.[1, 2] They also concluded that activation of deep muscles was necessary for spinal stability. Without this active muscular system supporting the spine, the passive joints themselves (which include the disc and the smaller facet joints) would crumble under the weight of just five to 10 pounds. So this active muscular system and its neural control system are critical to spinal health.

   How do these systems work together in practice? Imagine your spine as a crane or heavy earth-moving machine. When this machine has to move a heavy item from one area to another, it must first attach itself with extending footholds so that its base is stable before it can extend the arm of the crane in order to pull up a weight. This is similar to the system in your spine, where you need the smaller muscles to be active and working well to hold together the individual vertebrae. The longer muscles can then adequately propel the body forward or help lift an item off the floor.

Here is a way to gauge the strength of your stabilizing muscles: If you notice when you bend that you cannot bend fully, or if you experience a "hitch" that requires you to bend your hips or knees to complete the bend, you likely have a stability problem in your spine due to weakness of these stabilizing muscles.

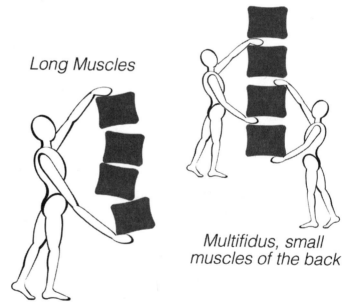

Long Muscles

Multifidus, small muscles of the back

The smaller muscles, such as the multifidus, act to stabilize vertebrae. These are selectively weakened in patients with back pain and with age. The longer muscles act to move the whole spine. When strengthening a painful spine, it is important to isolate the stabilizing muscle to prevent the longer muscles from doing all of the work.

People who need to improve their stability may also develop periodic spasms or find it difficult to sit or stand for longer periods of time. I have found that patients sometimes develop hip, knee, or shoulder pain in their attempt to compensate for the core weakness. Fortunately, all of these symptoms point to a deficit in stability that can be resolved through appropriate targeted strengthening.

As you age, however, these stability muscles can selectively weaken. They can also become weakened when you experience pain because you may consciously or unconsciously try to avoid using them. In any case, we can expect these deep stability muscles in our back to serve us well for bending and moving over a lifetime only if we ensure they stay strong.

We can expect these deep stability muscles in our back to serve us well for bending and moving over a lifetime only if we ensure they stay strong.

The other key muscles are the muscles around the abdomen, such as the oblique abdominal muscles and the transversus abdominis. These muscles act as a corset that helps to support the spine. Weight lifters use abdominal braces to prevent injury, and they are often prescribed for patients with back pain. Although I agree with the use of braces for weight lifters or for those whose jobs involve heavy lifting, these braces also weaken the key abdominal muscles and are not recommended for regular use.

178   TAKE BACK CONTROL

You may ask, "Well, what about the six-pack abdominal muscles (also called the rectus abdominis)? I thought those were key." Although I would still recommend strengthening these "mirror muscles"—so called because they, like the pectoral muscles in the chest and biceps in the arms, are the muscles people can see—ironically they are the least important in stabilizing the spine!

SPINE STABILIZATION 101

There are two types of exercises I *would* recommend for those with chronic low back pain—or for those who want to prevent it. These routines are good for kickstarting the activation of the dormant core muscles that support the spine.

1. **Activating the transversus abdominis (TA) and pelvic floor.** The TA creates a corset around your spine. It is hypoactive (underactive) in back pain patients and even in the majority of the population. Most people can barely suck in their stomach because of a lack of firing of this muscle.

   I find the easiest way to bring awareness to the TA is to turn onto your belly with your toes touching the floor and your elbows flexed at your side. Pull your belly button away from the floor. The muscle you feel contracting is the TA.

Turn on your back with your feet flat on the floor and your hips and knees flexed. Make sure that your pelvis is in a neutral position by arching it, then flattening it, and then find the midpoint. Now contract the same muscle you did while on your belly.

Firing the TA alone is not enough, since you need the pelvic floor to also engage. Now imagine yourself urinating and stopping yourself mid-flow. It's a gentile, upward lifting action. Simultaneously, fire the TA that you had brought awareness to.

To do these exercises, breathe normally, and activate the muscles for at least 5 seconds at a time for 10 repetitions. Repeat this process four times a day. Do this exercise for three weeks and you will notice a profound difference in your ability to maintain a flat lower abdomen.

Try using this muscle during functional activities. All you need to do is pull in your lower tummy like a greyhound whenever you bend over—whether you are brushing your teeth or picking up your young child. These muscles will now fire during your daily activities and protect your spine.

2. **Activating the multifidus.** Lie on your belly over a pillow. Push your right hip into the pillow. Try to bring awareness to the muscle that is contracting on the left lower back. If you can, reach back to feel the muscle

contract. Hold the contraction for 20 seconds; then do the other side. Try this exercise 10 times on each side.

For the next progression, raise up on "all fours," making sure that your hands are directly under the shoulders and the knees directly under the pelvis. Make sure that you are in a neutral position by rotating your pelvis both directions and finding the middle position. Place a thick magazine under your right knee. Next, lift your left knee and right hand to the same height as the magazine. As an optional progression of this exercise, you can extend your raised left leg back, and as a further step, raise your right arm in front of you, but make sure to keep the pelvis in the same neutral position.

For more on these home strengthening activities, visit www.takebackcontrol.com.

2. **The second reason most people have suboptimal back strength is that with traditional core exercises, it's difficult to control the resistance through the entire range of motion and to sequentially apply a measurable, heavier resistance.**

Planking, for example, even though I like it, strengthens the muscle at only one position.

Many people think that their exercises sufficiently strengthen their core, but how can you know? Alex is not alone in having poor core strength despite doing all the standard core strengthening exercises.

The person who helped define normal back strength at different ranges of motion was Arthur Jones. Research funded by Arthur Jones at the University of Florida measured the isolated back strength of normal volunteers who did not have any back pain.

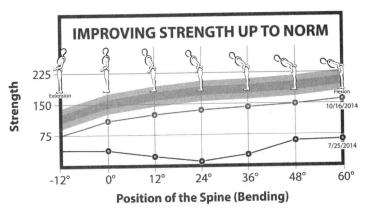

The shaded zone depicts the normal expected strength of the patient at different amounts of bending. This normal zone was developed by testing many patients, all with similar age and gender, who did not experience back pain. The 7/25/2014 graph is the strength of a patient with chronic back pain. The 10/16/2014 graph is the same patient after three months of specialized strengthening.

As you can see from the shaded zone on the graph, we naturally have more strength in our back muscles when we are bent forward (flexion). Also, there is a smooth transition of our strength between bending forward and standing upright, then bending back (extension). With chronic back pain, the graph can become uneven and indicate significantly lower levels in a person's strength (the 7/25/2014 graph). Doing core exercises in only one back position is just not adequate to bring this curve back to normal.

One solution is to do reverse sit-ups. These work well to strengthen the lower back through the entire range of motion. You can do this exercise by lying face down on a high bench and having someone hold your legs. Most large gyms have reverse sit-ups equipment, also called the Roman chair, that holds onto your lower extremities so you can do this exercise (see diagram).

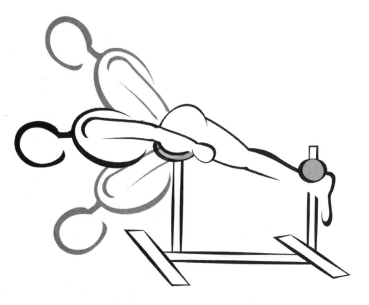

Roman chair exercise. This exercise helps strengthen the multifidus and other low back muscles. First, position yourself face down by placing the pads behind your ankles and in front of your pelvis. Then do a "reverse sit-up." To strengthen weakened spinal stabilization muscles, it is important not to use the gluteal muscles or hamstrings. (It's also important not to overextend since this can cause increased pain and use of non-spinal muscles.) Afterward, you should feel the burn in the muscles around your spine, not in your buttock or back of thighs.

I recommend doing 10 repetitions first with no added weight. This exercise is particularly beneficial because you can increase resistance and do so throughout the range of motion. The first modification is to do the exercise with the hands overhead. A further modification would be doing the exercise with a kettlebell to increase resistance. You can even strengthen your oblique muscles by positioning yourself on your side as a further modification. This is a great exercise you can do during your workouts to start combating core muscle weakness.

3. Sedentary lifestyles and bad posture can lead to permanent problems.

Postural problems are very common today. Thanks to the sedentary lifestyles that are now considered "normal" for most people, we spend much of our time with our bodies fixed in unhealthy positions. For example, eight hours of sitting at a desk puts the low back discs and muscles in a less than ideal position. Many hours of using our smartphones, as we discussed in Chapter 5 with the "text neck" epidemic, puts our head and neck in a suboptimal position. These positions cause us to forsake our natural center of gravity and can further affect the way we carry ourselves over time.

In fact, the key to reducing strain on all structures in the body is to generally place them in line with our center of gravity. Merriam-Webster defines "center of gravity" as the point at which the entire weight of a body may be thought of as centered so that if supported at this point the body would balance perfectly.

The key to reducing strain is to align with our center of gravity.

When we maintain ourselves in this balanced position, the least amount of effort is needed, and the least amount of force is placed on our tissues. This means that when viewed from the side, a gravity line should intersect the ear, shoulder, hip, knee, and ankle. When viewed from the front or back, you can draw a line right down the center of the body and both sides would look identical. The shoulders and pelvis are level.

Consider the Leaning Tower of Pisa. Now that it is leaning, there is much more strain on its foundation, and it will only relentlessly continue to bend until it fully fails, unless more is done to shore up its foundation. Actually, the tower has been leaning so long—almost 840 years now—that it's tempting to believe it will never fall. But the truth is that ever since it first began to lean during construction (as the foundation settled unevenly in the soft soil), there have been hundreds of interventions to keep it from falling. These included building compensations on one side of the tower and numerous adjustments by engineers over the years. However, the sad reality remains that the 12th century masonry, which has absorbed hundreds of years of excess stress due to leaning, could crumble at any time and completely collapse the tower. Even a minor earthquake could spell its end despite these heroic efforts.[3]

Building on a poor foundation (poor posture) can have similarly catastrophic results for the back. Scientists have studied the pressure as seen inside the disc of the low back when individuals stand in different positions. The results are astonishing because they demonstrate the tremendous difference—for better or for worse—that slight shifts in posture make.

Studies have been performed to assess the pressure within a disc during different postures.[4,5] Compared to someone standing in a relaxed standing pose, a person who has even a slight bend in her back creates *four and one half* times more pressure inside the disc when she lifts a pre-defined weight. However, if she lifts correctly with her legs, the pressure decreases to just three times as much, and only twice as much if she holds the weight close to her body.

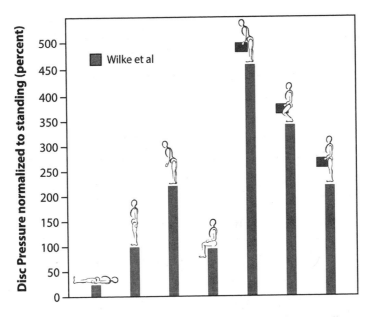

Maintaining a correct posture and lifting correctly dramatically reduce pressure on the discs of the spine.

Even without lifting anything, a simple forward bend results in two to two and a half times increase in the disc pressure. And if you are sitting in a forward slouched position, you are putting two and a half times more pressure on the disc than when you stand upright. In contrast, lying down causes only a 20 percent strain in the disc when compared to standing. This is why most back pain patients with disc abnormalities prefer to lie down when they are in a lot of pain.

So it's clear that your center of gravity makes a big difference in terms of strain on your discs. By becoming more aware of these differences and choosing postures that reduce strain in your daily activities, you can make a significant difference to your back health. While your disc does have some ability to heal itself as we have seen, you can improve its chances of remaining healthy by limiting this type of stress due to poor postures.

> *Your center of gravity makes a big difference in terms of strain on your discs.*

Also, when we strain, we significantly increase disc pressure. In fact, a simple sneeze or cough creates twice as much pressure as when we are at rest. Over the years, I've met many patients who have recounted an onset of severe sciatica or who have developed a disc herniation after a simple sneeze while they were sitting in a poor posture. (An easy way to protect yourself: If you're going to sneeze, make sure you're not in an awkward posture and brace yourself.)

Compensation Eventually Leads to Asymmetry...

I've had the opportunity to observe hundreds of patients' postures in our rehabilitation program and review countless posture pictures with a grid placed over the body to identify asymmetries. I'm still surprised at how often patients don't recognize the postural compensations they make. It's common, for example, to note one shoulder higher than the other, an asymmetric pelvis, a forward stoop, or even a bend to the side in patients.

This occurs due to our bodies' natural compensation mechanisms. Patients with disc herniations will frequently unknowingly lean away from the side of their disc herniation or sciatica to open up the space where the nerve exits. While these compensations are unconscious, they have a profound impact on unbalancing our center of gravity and contributing to further strain and injury in our backs. Our bodies can tolerate some of these minor asymmetries, but just like the Leaning Tower of Pisa, the compensation mechanism puts certain structures at increased strain so even more heroic attempts need to be made to shore up and maintain the abnormal posture.

Often, even after the disc herniation has gone away, patients will continue with these kinds of postural deficits since they have been accustomed to them, resulting in asymmetric wear of the disc and worsening disc degeneration. I have seen this particularly in patients who undergo scoliosis surgery or surgery for kyphosis (a forward bend of the spine). Even though their post-operative spinal alignment is excellent, their muscle memory and former habits result in a return of the same postural deficit.

These subtle differences in symmetry are not always visible in a mirror, unless you overlay a grid, or are accustomed to looking at postures frequently. This is why in our clinics, we take posture pictures of each new patient, overlay the grid and then review our findings with the patient.

You can do this for yourself at home. First put on form-fitting clothing and stand barefooted. Close your eyes and march slowly in place a few times. This allows your shoulders, pelvis, and feet to find their natural position. Have a friend take your picture from the front, side, and behind. You can use these pictures, or download one of the commonly available cell phone apps for posture. (I like the Posture Screen app, but there are many. Just search "posture.") Then monitor your posture over time to see if you are improving it.

I have seen many patients whose family members will tell me, "Aunt Millie is frequently a bit bent over to the right side...She's been that way for years, but only recently experienced severe leg pain." This posture may have started with poor positioning at a desk job decades earlier. In such cases, the current scans do show a predictable and corresponding abnormality that is consistent with these postural deficits.

For example, she may develop a degenerative scoliosis (because she leans to the side and rotates to write with her left hand) and compress the nerves on the concavity of the curve. However, the question not yet answered by scientific studies is: *If Aunt Millie's posture had been corrected many years ago, could she be symptom-free today?* My gut instinct tells me the answer to that question is yes.

...Soft Tissues and Ligaments Suffer Over Time...

Discs are not the only structures that are affected by bad posture. When soft tissues such as ligaments or tendons are exposed to a sustained load in a single direction without interruption—such as when you are sitting for several hours slumped at your desk—they can become stretched.

> *When soft tissues are exposed to a sustained load in a single direction without interruption, they can become stretched.*

This slight elongation, known as "creep," occurs naturally, and thereby allows the soft tissue to tolerate an increased load. The tough fibers within the soft tissues are rearranged, and when that occurs, the water content gradually gets squeezed from the soft tissues in these areas of sustained loading.

What are the consequences of this abnormal loading? If this load is not too excessive, soft tissues quickly recover and normalize to their original length. In the example above, if you slump at your desk, the soft tissues will still recover if you take frequent breaks and move around. (And remember the tips on sitting found in Chapter 2.) But when the load is too great, or even if there is limited interruption (i.e., you still spend many hours in a slumped position), the mechanical properties of soft tissues like ligaments and tendons can become altered.

These soft tissues can then become very susceptible to failure or can develop small microfractures when fatigued—even with normal loads—which results in pain, even when there is no obvious trauma. Sometimes even a minor trauma—like bending to lift a piece of trash or to brush your teeth—can bring on an episode of severe back pain. I have many patients who can attest to this.

...and the Patient Now Needs Surgery That Could Have Been Avoided.

Sustained poor posture not only results in the soft tissues being more susceptible to injury. Over time, these postural abnormalities can progress and result in a rigid deformity that is difficult to treat even with surgery. To change the alignment of a rigid, deformed spine, a surgeon may need to essentially cut a wedge out of the spine in order to realign it. The surgery also requires holding the spine with screws at multiple points of fixation and fusing it. And unfortunately, fusing multiple levels of the spine does result in increased strain at the adjacent discs above and below the fusion.

When discs surrounding a fusion prematurely degenerate, it is called "adjacent disc disease." If you imagine the spine as a chain with multiple links, when many of these links are welded together, the remaining links in the chain need to pick up the slack and therefore experience a lot more pressure with movement.

This can cause the adjacent discs to fail prematurely and either degenerate or become unstable. It's a very common consequence of spinal fusion surgery that is quite vexing for patients and surgeons. Such operations also result in significant blood loss if they are performed as open surgeries. (There are minimally invasive options that result in less blood loss, but may not be as effective for correcting severe deformities.)

Wouldn't you prefer to correct your posture naturally? If you begin correcting your posture today, you can undo much of the damage it has likely sustained to this point. Don't wait, because each day that you don't allow your alignment to stem from your center of gravity, you are adding a degree of pressure to a spine that desperately wants to serve you better.

The wonderful news is that you don't need an MRI scan, an X-ray, or knowledge of the underlying pathology or anatomy to correct many postural problems. Simple astute observation, stretching and strengthening, and body awareness work well. A simple way for us to keep the forces evenly distributed to our spine is not to load one side of our body more than the other. For example, consider women who wear a purse on one side of the body or across their neck…or children and teenagers who carry a heavy backpack on one side of the body to ensure they don't look "uncool." It's the nervous system that compensates to maintain balance in spite of the uneven weight distribution by shifting the rest of the body parts (head, pelvis, shoulders) in order to keep alignment.

Think about the position a man is in when he places his bulky wallet in a back pants pocket and then sits on that bulge in an office chair all day. Because his pelvis is tilted to one side, his spine needs to tilt and rotate the other direction in order to keep his head above his pelvis. In this way, his shoulders and head position compensate and act as a counterbalance. Unfortunately, this chain of events (that results from placing a wallet in the pocket) will have an unintended consequence over time. Individuals who chronically keep a thick wallet in that same back pocket will likely develop upper back or neck pain, and may never correlate it to this habit.

To avoid these kinds of compensations, it's important that weight is distributed evenly on both sides of the body and asymmetric positions are not maintained for long periods of time. Otherwise, there will be a compensatory shift in the position of the spine and trunk that may cause pain that is not easily attributable to these subtle habits. Anyone carrying purses or satchels should try to cross them over their bodies to better distribute the weight. Men should try to keep their wallets as thin as possible, and should be sure to remove and store them either in their front pocket or somewhere safe. Finally, parents need to encourage children to wear their backpacks "correctly," with one strap on each shoulder.

It is particularly important that children develop good postural habits with respect to how they carry weight since their spines are still developing. In a developing spine, poor posture and the resulting mismatched forces can result in growth that is also uneven. This "remodeling" of the spine occurs because loading of a growth plate alters growth in a predictable manner: Compression (pushing together) decreases growth while "distraction" (pulling apart) increases growth.

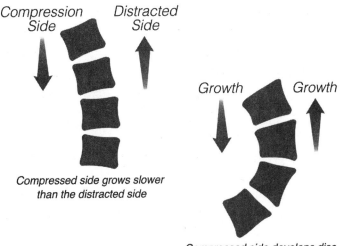

Compression Side

Distracted Side

Growth

Growth

Compressed side grows slower than the distracted side

Compressed side develops disc degeneration and collapses further

In a growing spine, uneven forces result in uneven growth. If the spine is maintained in a side bending position as on the left image, the left side of the vertebrae (in the concavity) doesn't grow as much as the right side (the convexity). This results in worsening of the curve as shown in the right image, as the faster growing portion of the spine twists around the slower growing portions.

We counter these asymmetric forces for advantage when treating scoliosis patients. By bracing the spine during growth, we can redistribute the force more evenly on the vertebrae and disc and thereby prevent worsening of the deformity. By the same reasoning, if we asymmetrically load the spine in a growing patient, we may be causing permanent spinal deformities. The take-home lesson: The spine is inherently "moldable"...for better or for worse.

The spine is inherently "moldable"...
for better or for worse.

EXAMPLES OF TIGHT MUSCLES AND TENDONS

While strengthening usually results in the shortening of muscles, flexibility lengthens them again to maintain balance. That's why flexibility is critical to any treatment program for the spine. If you were to only strengthen the "mirror muscles" in the front that people see (specifically, the pectoral muscles in the chest and biceps in the arms), then your shoulders would rotate forward as a result of the shortening of these muscles.

Consequently, you could end up with shoulder pain from increased irritation of the rotator cuff. Also, the nerves and blood vessels going down the arm could get compressed due to the shortened muscles, causing arm pain and numbness (also called "thoracic outlet syndrome"). The forward leaning posture could also lead to disc herniations in the neck and low back. That's why it is so important to stretch those front muscles after strengthening them. In this way, you maintain correct posture and balance.

Another example of how muscle tightness can result in injury is the iliopsoas muscle. This is a muscle group that lifts up the hip. Since this muscle is a primary "fight or flight muscle," it is affected by stress. As you can imagine, the first thing you would do when running away from danger is to flex your hip and pull your leg towards your chest to initiate running. As a result, this muscle can hold a lot of emotionally charged tension.

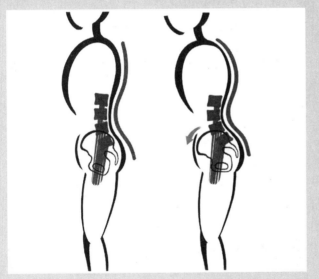

On the left is a normal spine. On the right, when the iliopsoas muscle becomes tight and shortened, the spine becomes "hyperlordotic," or abnormally curved, which causes pain.

Prolonged sitting—at a desk or driving in a car, for example—also shortens this muscle. Any time it becomes tight, it rotates the pelvis forward and in turn results in increasing the curvature of the low back. As a result, a person can begin to experience an ache in the lower back, which can spread throughout the back and hips. It can even cause pain as you rise up out of a seated position or stand upright too quickly. (This is also why patients with a tight iliopsoas muscle frequently experience pain in the second half of a sit-up.)

To avoid this kind of pain, it's important that any strengthening program identifies tightness where it is present and adequately stretches out the iliopsoas, the hamstrings, and the adductor muscles of the hip. The same is true for the upper trunk; the front chest muscles must be stretched out well and the shoulder blades lowered and brought together. (You can do this at home with a simple door stretch by extending your arms as you walk through it. Continue to walk forward until you feel a stretch within the chest.)

Any strengthening program must also identify tightness where it is present and stretch out the iliopsoas, hamstrings, and adductor muscles.

There are multiple deviations that can commonly occur to your posture. Each deviation results in corresponding imbalanced muscle activity (either over- or underactive muscles) or tight soft tissues such as tendons or muscles. Each deviation can therefore be addressed by specific strengthening exercises and stretches. The description of each of these is beyond the scope of this book, but can be found at www. takebackcontrol.com or www.bodybuilding. com/fun/posture-power-how-to-correct-your-body-alignment.html.

4. **It takes hard work to build up muscle.**

While our ancestors lived a lifestyle that naturally required regular physical activity during their days—bending, lifting, and moving—most of us today experience a more sedentary way of life. If you do not engage in daily activities that naturally load these muscles, they will atrophy. So you must actively strengthen them.

In years past, physicians advised patients with back pain to take it easy. But as we saw in Chapter 5, prolonged rest or decreased activity can actually hinder rather than help back pain. Weak back muscles that become deconditioned through further lack of use cause even more problems for patients. In fact, in one newer trend, some physicians are going so far as to prescribe patients to use "aggressive rehabilitation" through intensive exercise to overcome chronic back pain.[6] While it may sound counterintuitive to intentionally stress a bad back, the truth is that building up these muscles can provide what seems like a miracle cure for some patients.

Even if you don't have a bad back, effective strengthening can help reduce the natural loss of muscle as you age. Between ages 50 to 70, we can lose up to 40 percent of our muscle and 30 percent of our strength, making us more vulnerable to balance problems that can cause falls. Many believe that weakened muscles contribute and in fact may be critical to developing chronic back pain. High-intensity resistance training two to three times per week will also reduce arthritis pain, improve mobility and daily functions (like walking, climbing stairs, or getting out of a chair), and lower your risk of heart disease and stroke.[7]

How Does Exercise Enhance Strength?

So now that we see how important weakness is in developing pain, it becomes apparent that training and exercise are the clear solutions. How does exercise work? There are two main mechanisms at play—one involving the nerves and one involving the muscles.[8]

The neural basis of muscle strengthening involves the ability to recruit more muscle cells in a simultaneous manner. There is a natural response of the nervous system to keep muscles from overworking and possibly ripping apart as it creates a level of force to which it is not accustomed. Training decreases this inhibitory response or "brake" that the nervous system applies. Also, untrained muscles tend not to fire together. As you can imagine, having the muscles fire in unison will increase their function.

Exercise can result in significant gains in strength, even without building new muscle, by training the nerves to stop inhibiting and to synchronize their firing. This nerve response is responsible for much of the strength gains seen in the initial stages of all strength training and in women and adolescents who gain strength without bulking up.

The muscle response to exercise is a much slower process and depends on the creation of new muscle proteins, which results in enlargement, or hypertrophy, of the cells.

To develop more muscle, be prepared for hard work and slow gains. In fact, the body will build muscle only in response to a combination of progressive resistance training, proper diet, and adequate rest. Here's why: Resistance causes stress, which first breaks down muscles. With appropriate diet and rest, the muscles then grow as an "over-compensation" type of mechanism to protect the body from future stress.

The human body breaks down and rebuilds muscles over a several-day period. In fact, this rebuilding peaks about 24 to 36 hours after training and continues at an increased rate for up to as much as 72 hours. So adequate rest between training sessions is a key ingredient for building muscle. You must first stress the muscles enough to "damage" them and then allow a sufficient amount of time between exercises in order for the muscle to rebuild enough. Otherwise, you will simply continue to break down muscle for poor results.

Applying adequate stress to each of your target muscles is important so that it leads to an increase in the release of hormones and greater flow of nutrients into the muscles. The important thing to understand here is that when you lift a light weight, it doesn't involve a slight effort on the part of *all* of your biceps muscle fibers. Rather, only a few fibers—just the exact number required to perform that particular movement—will be involved and only they will be working to their limit while the other muscles will remain inactive.

During this lighter lifting activity, while the rest of the fibers (the other non-working fibers) may get passively pushed, pulled, or moved about by the movement, they will contribute absolutely nothing to the work being performed. As a result, unless you are working all or at least most of your muscle fibers and breaking them all down, they will not build up as quickly as you would like. The resistance must be heavy enough and throughout the range of motion for all of the muscle fibers to be affected. The exercise must therefore be "high intensity."

The Benefits of High Intensity Training

At the encouragement of my mentor, Dr. Mooney, I began to study work by Arthur Jones, a pioneer in high intensity training (HIT), a training style where exercises are brief, infrequent, and intense. HIT proponents like Jones believe that this approach is superior for strength and size building compared to other methods. Advocates also stress the importance of controlled lifting speeds and strict form, to avoid bouncing and jerking, which can cause injury and compromise results.

The whole idea in HIT is to be as efficient and targeted as possible in your workout to get the best results in the shortest amount of time. As someone who believed in the value of measuring one's progress, Jones did extensive studies to evaluate the effectiveness of various methods to improve strength efficiently.

The whole idea in HIT is to be as efficient and targeted as possible in your workout to get the best results in the shortest amount of time.

One such technique he studied was the impact of "negative repetitions" on strength building. This is a training technique where, for example, you would start with your chin above a pull-up bar and slowly lower yourself down. This is the "negative" of the normal movement (because we can lower a far greater weight than we can pull up).

He also studied the value of "static holding," where an individual holds weight with muscles fully contracted for up to 30 seconds.

The goal with both of these exercise techniques is to exhaust the muscle thoroughly to promote "hypertrophy," the process whereby muscles break down and then rebuild. This stimulates further muscle growth and greater strength. Muscles are weakest in certain motions that involve "positive" or "contracting" movements. For example, when you raise your arm during a biceps curl, the muscle shortens and this is a positive contraction. A negative contraction is when you are lowering that same weight, as we discussed above with respect to negative repetitions. Try doing negative contractions at the gym to get a feel for how much more the muscle is worked.

Three different approaches can be utilized to thoroughly exhaust or exercise a muscle: repetition at a heavy weight, statically holding a weight at different angles, and lowering a weight at a slow, controlled speed. Repetition at heavy weight is great for building muscle, but puts a lot of strain on the joints.

Although you may not be able to lift a weight for one more repetition, you will certainly be able to hold it statically for a period of time. This can help make up for using less weight. Another commonly used technique is lifting a lower weight at slow and controlled speed. Body builders commonly use these different methods for excellent results. While standard HIT worked well for the body builders of the time, there are many of these same principles that can be applied to patients with core muscle weakness and chronic back and neck pain.

While there are different techniques for muscle building, one common agreement is that it is important to measure baseline strength, gradually increase resistance, and assess effectiveness. Also, there is no way to "comfortably" build up muscle; it has to be done with enough intensity to truly stress the muscle. Building up muscle occurs by applying this stress—via exercise—to your muscles, and then allowing your body to adapt to this stress by providing it with adequate nutrition and rest. All said, it is a consistent cycle of stress and adaptation.

THE PROS AND CONS OF POPULAR HIGH INTENSITY INTERVAL TRAINING (HIIT) EXERCISE PROGRAMS

One of the most popular high intensity interval exercise programs is CrossFit. Others include P90X and Insanity. CrossFit is a demanding fitness program crossing many different types of functional movements and workout regimens such as mixed martial arts, running, powerlifting, and gymnastics in order to promote core strength, aerobic fitness, and comprehensive total-body conditioning.

Note that for HIIT workouts the premise is to efficiently burn as many calories as possible in the least amount of time. Note that these are different from the HIT (with one "I") workouts that seek to build muscles by maximizing the stress placed on them.

The goal is not to lift the most or be the fastest or to master any one exercise, but to learn a broad cross section of lifts and exercises so as to be fit in all ways and prepared for any type of movement. The program uses whiteboards as a scoreboard to keep accurate scores and records, runs a clock, and uses the fostered sense of community to harness camaraderie, competition, and fun.

My personal experience with CrossFit is that it is effective for general conditioning. I am concerned, however, since I see a disproportionate number of young patients who have developed disc herniations after the exercises. This usually has occurred after multiple sets, and I can almost always trace the injury to bad form in a fatigued person. Since CrossFit is so popular, this increased incidence of disc herniations may not be an aberration. I would, however, suggest that even for healthy individuals, it is very important to maintain good form during the exercises. It is important not to sacrifice technique for intensity.

For patients with significant back or neck pain or nerve impingement, however, I would not recommend starting with CrossFit. Most patients with chronic spinal pain have imbalance in their muscle strength and activation, making the complex exercises used in CrossFit more likely to cause symptoms. Often, to get better at complex functional movements, it is important to improve strength with basic movements as well. It is much better to equalize those muscle imbalances using the principles of high intensity training, but in an isolated and therefore safer way.

Sometimes We Need Sustained, Supervised "Medical Exercise"

Many years ago, my mentor in non-operative treatment, Dr. Vert Mooney, believed that as spine surgeons we needed to be much more involved with non-operative care in general and therapeutic exercise in particular. He was a believer in not only high intensity training, but inclusion of exercise in medical treatment similar to how we dose medication that we prescribe and measure its effect. He introduced me to the work of Arthur Jones and MedX medical exercise equipment. This equipment isolates the back muscles, allows strengthening throughout the range of motion, and is the most scientifically studied.

An important difference between Arthur Jones and his predecessors (as well as others who currently treat back pain through strengthening) is that Jones developed ways to isolate the spinal muscles and strengthen the stabilizing muscles by safely ratcheting up the stress on the muscle. The key to this isolation is to immobilize the pelvis while doing back strengthening. If the pelvis is free to move, the spinal muscles don't have to contract to extend the spine.

In back pain patients, this isolation is much better accomplished through the use of machine-based stabilization exercises. This approach allows us to easily increase the resistance on isolated muscles incrementally, which results in improved muscle stimulation and growth of these inhibited muscles. The strengthening is done throughout the range of motion, which as described above has a profound impact on activities. These factors were missing in Alex's training regimen.

Also, free weight exercises can result in more strain on unstable spinal joints than do machine-stabilized exercises. Even though Alex had all of the motivation in the world, the standard exercises caused him pain. When patients are secured in machines similar to the

MedX and the types we have in our SpineZone clinics, even those with debilitating pain who didn't feel that they could exercise can sense the confidence to start moving and strengthening.

Machine-based exercises also have the advantage of being standardized. Even though Alex's professional travel schedule forced him to visit different clinics and different practitioners, we could gauge his progress similarly to how an X-ray taken in San Diego can be read in New York City. We could observe both the sequential improvement of his ability to lift more as well as the normalization of strength compared to patients without pain. Our goal with spinal rehabilitation in general and with the SpineZone clinics in particular is to have a consistent non-operative treatment that, not unlike a prescription pill, can be counted on for its consistent dosages and effects.

> *Our goal with spinal rehabilitation is to have a consistent non-operative treatment that, not unlike a prescription pill, can be counted on for its consistent dosages and effects.*

Quantitating exercise treatment is a key element in any back rehabilitation program. Upon seeing the incremental improvement in strength, patients are empowered because they can experience the capabilities of their bodies first-hand. We have seen that as patients regain their expected normal strength and normalize their posture, their pain subsides.

In a setting where there is a deep understanding of both non-operative and surgical spinal disease, exercise has many benefits. Many studies have noted that in addition to reducing pain and increasing strength, exercise can effectively reduce the behavioral, cognitive, and disability aspects of back pain.[9] In a medical setting in particular, exercise reduces disability by desensitizing a patient to unsubstantiated fears and pessimistic beliefs about pain.

In fact, in a recent review of patients who completed the SpineZone program from 10-01-15 to 03-31-16, anti-inflammatory usage decreased from 55 percent to 12 percent and narcotic usage from 34 percent to 11 percent. Over a two-year period, we showed over a 25 percent decrease in the rate of surgery. I am proud to say that we have made long-term changes in patients' outlook regarding their spine condition and activity levels.

Hopefully, this chapter has shown you the inherent value in working to undo much of the damage that your back has sustained due to injury or lifestyle. We have become conditioned to the idea that pills and surgery are the best solutions, but my team has proven that there is another way—a way that is safer and yields predictable results.

A holistic approach incorporates many aspects of care that, when taken one at a time, may seem less effective than the perceived quick fix of a pill or surgery— yet, actually, they are often far more successful.

As this chapter demonstrates, there are many factors to consider as you begin to develop a plan to get "stronger and straighter" to fully rehabilitate your back. You must ensure you take into account the need for stability, posture, musculature, flexibility, and the nervous system to lay a strong foundation and also hold realistic expectations of the many treatment options available to you. This can be a challenging process, particularly if you are struggling with a long-term imbalance that you have developed over many years. But by acting proactively early on—before you develop serious symptoms—you can avoid long-term problems and enjoy a lifetime free from pain.

If you would like to view a comprehensive list of exercises that can further strengthen the muscles supporting your spine, please visit www. takebackcontrol.com.

Key Learning Points: Getting Stronger and Straighter

1. There are four main reasons why people do not have optimal back strength: the main stabilizing muscles of the spine become weakened with age; standard core exercises cannot control the resistance through the entire range of motion and cannot sequentially apply a measureable, heavy resistance; many people lead sedentary lifestyles and/or have spine-weakening bad posture; it takes hard work to build muscle.

2. Muscle strengthening is best performed by isolating the muscle, exercising all of its fibers, gradually increasing the resistance over time, and measuring progress. Rest and good nutrition between training sessions are vital for maximal muscle growth.

3. An effective program to treat back pain acknowledges and addresses the important roles played by stability, center of gravity, muscle anatomy, the nervous system, and flexibility.

4. To strengthen the core, a training program must address not just the abdominal muscles, but more importantly, the stabilizing back and flank muscles. This can be difficult to accomplish at home without appropriate equipment to isolate these muscles, and as such, sometimes supervised medical exercise is necessary.

5. Exercise performed correctly is empowering since we can experience the capabilities of our bodies first-hand. This is the best remedy against our fear when we have pain.

CHAPTER 7

THE IMPACT OF HABITS

> "We are what we repeatedly do."
>
> —Aristotle

In earlier chapters, we talked about the role of bad habits—texting, sitting, sedentary lifestyles, or driving with improper posture—in contributing to the epidemic of back and neck pain. If *good* postural habits and routines are vital to relieving our pain, what is the best way to form them? How can we use the habit-making process to our advantage when we have a chronic neck or back condition?

William James, an American philosopher and psychologist, once wrote, "Could the young but realize how soon they will become mere walking bundles of habits, they would give more heed to their conduct while in the plastic state." He clearly understood the value of cultivating healthy habits.

But it takes time to change one's daily routine, so it's important to cultivate patience on this journey. To implement real change, habits need to be "hardwired" so that they are automatic. Likewise, the benefit of good posture and strength comes only with sustained practice for any lasting benefit.

> *To implement real change, habits need to be "hardwired" so that they are automatic.*

Achieving "Automaticity" in Your Habits

So, what does science say about habits? A study done at the University College London reported that, on average, 66 days were needed to create a new habit, but this also ranged from 18 to 254 days to reach a 95 percent "automaticity"...In other words, to act without thinking.[1] This notion of automaticity turns out to be a central driver for habits. However, it's important not to misinterpret findings. The study also showed that missing one opportunity to perform a behavior does not materially affect the habit formation process. It is okay, therefore, to mess up every now and then because building better habits is not an all or nothing process.

The Three Fundamental Phases of Habit Forming

Many years ago, a cosmetic surgeon, Dr. Maxwell Maltz, popularized the thinking that it could take only 21 days to develop a new habit. But actually, this 21-day myth began as a misinterpretation of his findings regarding improving self-image. Even though his findings applied to a very specific instance, the idea that it could apply to all new habits took off and is quoted often.

A different basis for developing sustainable positive habits was identified by Tom Bartow, a man who successfully started an advanced training program for investing firm Edward Jones. Bartow describes three phases of habit formation: The "honeymoon" phase is the first phase and is usually the result of something that is inspiring change, such as a New Year's resolution, an episode of pain, or an appealing image of yourself that you would like to adopt.

However, the key to hardwiring change actually comes in the next two phases. The "fight-through phase" is phase two, where one recognizes the scope of the problem. A person essentially asks, "What would happen if I create this new habit?" and conversely, "What would happen—what emotions would I feel—if I didn't change my habit or reach this goal?"

In this fight-through phase, it is important to project what would happen (using great detail) in the next five years if you do not begin to make these changes. To turn the impetus of the honeymoon intent into a sustainable habit, it's important that you win at least two or three of these "fight-throughs" to convince yourself that change is needed. The key is to reach stage three where the habit has become "second nature"; it is ingrained and hardwired.

The Importance of Fighting Through Setbacks

However, even after a new habit has become second nature, it's easy to experience an interruption due to a long vacation, illness, or even a long weekend. These interruptions can send you back to the fight-through phase. And yet, once you win two or three fight-through rounds, you'll be back to where the habit is second nature. The key is to avoid the discouragement monster where you think thoughts like, *This isn't working and there is nothing I can do.*

It's also important not to stop short. If you do experience early success, don't be lured in by the seduction of success, where you are tempted to think you are special, in that you can continue to experience the same great results while shortcutting processes that work. When you experience what seems like a "quick fix," it can deter you from developing long-term habits that sustain your gains.[2]

Coincidentally, the time it takes to create a new habit is similar to the time it takes to restore back strength. As we discussed, muscles require time to hypertrophy, or enlarge, and therefore become stronger. With appropriate exercise and rest, it takes at least six to eight weeks to see noticeable changes in muscle and strength and up to twelve weeks to achieve significant changes. Because the timeframe for gaining strength is similar to that of forming habits, it has served us well in our Spine-Zone clinics. In the amount of time it takes us to restore back strength, we are also able to instill a change in the very habits that will keep those muscles strong.

With appropriate exercise and rest,
it takes at least six to eight weeks to
see noticeable changes in muscle and
strength and up to twelve weeks to
achieve significant changes.

In this chapter I will explain how the SpineZone team helps patients overcome the obstacles and mindsets that so often delay patients' healing.

Fixing Your Posture Takes Time

It's perhaps not surprising that it also takes time to make lasting changes in one's postural habits and work ergonomics. It takes time to unlearn and relearn so many of the subconscious habits that frequently result in back strain, such as the way we bend, the way we twist, the way we lift things off the ground, and the way we place things on a shelf. Each of these habits can impact the stress that the spine absorbs.

In addition, if we have established postural deficits due to longstanding symptoms or habits—ways we compensate for pain or ways in which our work desk is configured, for example—it will take time to develop true body awareness to change these. Because we have learned that the commitment to at least a 10-week program significantly improves patient outcomes, we have partnered with physician groups to ensure patients can take advantage of an uninterrupted 10-week treatment period. (This is in contrast to most authorization for therapies, which is typically much shorter and therefore not well suited to meaningfully altering long-term habits.)

We've also found that patients ask for and benefit significantly when they can engage in a monthly maintenance program once to twice per month following their initial 10-week treatment period, to ensure their good habits remain second-nature to prevent long-term problems. In fact, more than 25 percent of our patients are willing to pay out-of-pocket—outside their insurance coverage—to do this type of long-term maintenance because they have experienced how effective it is.

The Best Way to Change Your Habits Is to Control Your Environment

We are more reliant on our environment—rather than our intentions—to trigger our actions and habits. Therefore, in order to radically change your behavior, it is important to first radically change your environment. It would be nice to think that we make our own choices and follow through on them, but we are actually very influenced by the things around us.

In the conclusion of his study on visual cues of portion size, Brian Wansink states, "using smaller than normal size plates, bowls, and glasses might lead people to believe that they had a full portion and make them less likely to ask for an extra (compensating) serving. Similarly, bulk snack products that are repackaged by a watchful parent into small portions and sealed into zip-lock baggies may provide the visual cue that leads a child to believe he or she has had a full serving of a snack when it was actually a fraction of what they might typically eat."[3]

If your environment dictates your actions, then you can use your environment to change your behavior. For example, spend time and effort making it easy to form good habits and take steps to make bad habits difficult to engage in.

When your motivation is high (for example, just after eating a big meal or the night before you plan to go to the gym), make sure to pack your gym clothes in a bag and place them in your car. If you are going to physical therapy, make multiple appointments in the future at the same time to eliminate the choices and guarantee that you keep your appointment. Similarly, your home exercise regimen should have clear implementation intentions, such as knowing where and when you will exercise.

In fact, in a study published in the *British Journal of Health Psychology,* participants who used these implementation intentions (they wrote down exactly when and where they would exercise each week) ended up following through with exercise at least one time per week 91 percent of the time compared to 38 percent follow-through in the control group. Interestingly, those who read motivational material about exercise, but did not plan, showed no increase in exercise compared to the control group.[4]

Try scheduling tasks during the same time in your daily schedule, including exercise. For example, do certain vital spine exercises—like the transverse abdominis activation from Chapter 6—at the same time every day, like before your lunch break or as soon as you wake up.

Six Tips for Forming—and Sustaining—Positive Habits[5]

With these ideas in mind, let's consider the best ways to ensure you develop habits that stick as you work to become stronger and straighter. The following six tips are courtesy of the U.S. Defense Centers of Excellence for Psychological Health & Traumatic Brain Injury. These tips are supported by research on how our brain motivates us to habituate new behaviors. Below, I explore each tip and put it in a "back pain treatment" context.

1. **Link the new behavior to a routine or environmental cue.** Sometimes people think that willpower is the key to adopting new habits and breaking bad ones. But actually, recent research shows that strength of will is just part of the answer, and habits can be used to prompt behavior. In his book *The Power of Habit*, Charles Duhigg describes a "habit loop model" that links a new routine to certain times of day or in response to specific cues.[6]

   In fact, Starbucks was able to effectively counter the tendency of its teenage employees to fall apart in the face of angry customers by instituting a new routine where baristas automatically repeated every customer order, explained that an order had been entered, and politely thanked customers. By using each new customer as a reminder for the routine, servers essentially adopted a new and automated routine that ensured courtesy and politeness to customers and replaced the tendency to respond rudely to unhappy or unfriendly customers.

I have found that a standard doorframe can serve as just such a cue for my patients who suffer from neck and upper back pain, tightness, and poor posture. By placing their hands on the side of the doorframe as they advance their chest through the threshold, they can stretch a tight chest and reposition their shoulders in one easy movement. In time, as they invariably are reminded by the multiple doorframes they meet in the course of a day, they are rewarded with better posture and relief of pain in the neck, upper back, and arms.

2. **Reward yourself.** By linking the performance of a difficult task to a reward—an "if-then" plan—you can associate a new and possibly uncomfortable behavior with something positive that you like so that the difficult task becomes associated with pleasure. Research shows that this linking creates a positive feedback loop that ensures repetition of the new behavior in the future, thus creating a positive spiral of success.[7] So put your thinking cap on: What would you enjoy for a job well done?

For many of my patients, timing the stretches they do at home to TV commercials seems to work well, with the viewing of a favorite TV show or sports event serving as the reward factor. There are usually at least four commercial breaks per hour, each lasting at least three to four minutes. By integrating home exercises and stretching routines into TV watching, it's efficient and easy to get it done consistently.

For example, I find that alternating strengthening (crunches, transverse abdominis activation, the superman pose, oblique abdominal strengtheners, and isometric neck exercises) and stretching (hamstring, adductors, anterior chest, neck, bridges, and hip flexors) at each commercial break is easily tolerated and seems to work well. Please visit www. takebackcontrol.com for details on these stretches and exercises.

3. **Repeat new behaviors and keep track of progress.** While repeating a behavior increases the likelihood for developing a new habit, research shows that what helps even more is to log how many times you perform the new behavior and if you are successful.[8,9] In one study on obesity, college students were asked to repeat a behavior daily, then log on to a website to report whether they performed the behavior, and also self-report how automatic the behavior had become. The average time until the habit became automatic was 66 days. (This study also confirmed that occasionally missing a day did not seem to affect the final outcome of the habit forming at 66 days.)[10] Applications such as Nike Training Club or the activity application on iPhones are good ways to log and track your exercises.

For patients who regularly visit our clinics, we promote participation in their home exercises and posture program, often using text reminders and phone calls for forward momentum. We have improved our compliance rate and have kept patients in the program longer with these tools. In fact, we believe that by developing a patient portal with enhanced digital monitoring techniques, we have significantly improved our patients' likelihood to "hardwire" new habits.

4. **Keep it simple.** In the same study, behaviors that were more complex were found to take longer to become habits. Stanford psychologist B.J. Fogg believes that tough habits stick when you can simplify behavior: "Goals are harmful unless they guide you to make specific behaviors easier to do. Don't focus your motivation on doing Behavior X. Instead, focus on making Behavior X easier to do." For those not accustomed to regular exercise and activity, waking up 20 minutes early or carving out time at lunch and simply adding a walk (either outside or treadmill) or bike ride (stationary or outside) will kick-start the process.

Once you get moving, it is important to add an element of strengthening to your routine. In patients unaccustomed to strength training, supervised high intensity exercise, performed for a short period of time only a few days a week, has resulted in large strength gains. At SpineZone, we've learned that patients are most compliant when they have a simple, effective, and focused spine strengthening session that is between 30 and 40 minutes and is sustained twice a week for 10 weeks.

Patients are most compliant when they have a simple, effective, and focused spine strengthening session that is between 30 and 40 minutes and is sustained twice a week for 10 weeks.

Similarly, by shortening and simplifying your gym workouts, you can increase the probability that you will comply with them. If performed with appropriate intensity, strength training can be very beneficial even when performed only once or twice a week.

As described in Chapter 6, using your gym's exercise machines with single sets and maximal intensity for up to 20 to 25 repetitions—or doing slow motion repetitions—are good ways to simplify your workout. These methods improve compliance, yet we are still able to incrementally increase the resistance to obtain the desired muscle growth and strength improvement.

5. **Make a detailed plan.** Just as you tend to lose weight when you have a weight loss goal or save more money when you have a budget, so too do you perform better when you have a plan or goal as you work to cultivate new habits. Studies show that making a goal-oriented habit will lead to more likely success than one that focuses on methods to create the new habit.[11] Our patients are asked which three functional goals are most important to them. By outlining a plan to restore normal strength, alignment, and flexibility, we pave a pathway for them to attain those specific goals. (This is called a patient-centered outcome, since the goal is defined by the patient and not by some arbitrary standard.)

I would suggest adopting the same strategy for yourself. Define three functional goals and break each into components. For example, if you want to be able to play tennis longer, you can separate the components that will help you attain your goal by improving your hip and knee strength, core rotational strength, and flexibility.

6. **Be accountable.** Research also shows that habits are most effective when they are announced to one or more people because these individuals can be a source of encouragement, motivation, or even create a little peer pressure to reinforce your new habit.[12] There are many ways to achieve this. You can talk with friends and family members, or seek out others who are also working on back strengthening for mutual accountability, perhaps even committing to a dedicated accountability buddy whom you check in with on a regular basis.

Pastor Rick Warren at Saddleback Church in Orange County, California, had great success teaching his parishioners a diet-lifestyle program using this principle. The psychiatrist Daniel Amen, who helped to develop the plan, explains that: "The secret sauce of Saddleback is we do this as a community. It's very different from most health plans where you do it with yourself and your wife. You get to do this with a whole community."[13]

Along the same lines, there is an old adage, "A problem shared is a problem halved." In a study published in the journal *Social Psychological and Personality Science,* researchers found that levels of stress hormones were significantly reduced when participants were able to vocalize how they felt about public speaking with others in the same situation.[14]

In this study, people discussed how they felt about public speaking with others who either felt the same way about public speaking (emotionally similar) or very different (emotionally dissimilar), while others were told not to discuss their feelings.

Interacting with emotionally similar participants decreased stress compared to not discussing fears. (Interestingly, interacting with a person who is emotionally dissimilar may actually be damaging to those who feel most threatened by the situation.)

At SpineZone, we have experienced the power of social networking and have adapted the concept to our cause. We've found that when patients suffer from similar problems in the same clinic, they can help each other gain confidence. Those who feel desperate and lonely in their battle with back pain are significantly helped by those who have successfully triumphed over their fear.

In addition to the natural encounters that happen between these patients in our clinics, we actively match patients with similar diagnoses and goals so they can help motivate each other, especially in the early stages of therapy when extra motivation is needed.

Motivation, Mindset, Measurement... and More

Empirically, I've noticed a few additional things in working with patients who are successful in creating good habits for back health. Patients who get great results are definitely those who are self-motivated. They believe in and feel empowered by their ability to regain long-term back health through the methods that we have explained to them. Undertaking the program is their decision—not someone else's—and they go into it believing that they can and will succeed.

Patients who can't let go of their belief that surgery is the ultimate fix or can't set aside catastrophic thinking often struggle to fully commit to a non-operative program in a way that will lead to success. So ask yourself before you begin: *Am I doing this for* me *or because my wife or doctor wants me to do it? Do I believe in the therapy program and am I committed to giving it my all? Or do I feel that all therapy is the same? Is there any way that I am sabotaging my chance for improvement?* Intrinsic motivation is important.

They also build on their success over time. It's important to establish a pattern of success as you build spine strength. When you see what you are accomplishing bit by bit, you become more likely to stick with a frequent strengthening schedule and more willing to increase training intensity. This is where measurement-driven rehabilitation is so important. (As business strategist H. James Harrington says, "Measurement is the first step that leads to control and eventually to improvement. If you can't measure something, you can't understand it. If you can't understand it, you can't control it. If you can't control it, you can't improve it.")

It's important to establish a pattern of success as you build spine strength.

For chronic and recurrent back pain, the best way to ensure you succeed is to take it slow. This is where a trainer can be particularly helpful by objectively assessing the strength of key muscles and designing a unique training program that is achievable for you and has a low likelihood of resulting in any worsening symptoms.

The point is to build your confidence through repeated successes and avoid the injuries and disappointment that come when we take on too much too fast. In the same way, it's useful to set a regular weekly routine so that you avoid the types of disruptions that we talked about earlier. Plan training sessions when possible for times when you feel your best rather than just hoping to fit it in.

And finally, silence your inner critic! Remember our earlier discussion of racing thoughts and how hard it can be to silence them? It's critical to master this skill to succeed at building new habits, particularly when it comes to learning new and unfamiliar postures. It's so easy to slip into thinking, *This therapy can't possibly fix my serious problem...I must be doing it wrong...It probably won't work...I'm never going to learn this!*

But remember that things that seem initially uncomfortable become more comfortable with practice. So while you are working on silencing your inner critic, use the opportunity to build a new and more nurturing voice. Replace negative thoughts with positive ideas that are reinforced by the facts of your successful rehabilitation like, *I must be building strength since I'm able to tolerate more resistance...Even though my pain still remains to some degree, I'm improving since I notice that I am able to function better...By keeping with it, I can unleash my body's self-healing capacity.*

The Importance of Social Support

In tip number six, we touched on the importance of accountability as a best practice to hardwire new habits. Intuitively, we all understand that a strong social network of supporters can help us keep on track when we are working on acquiring a new positive habit. It's much harder to stay on a healthy diet if your family isn't supportive. (Who can resist the aroma of freshly baked chocolate chip cookies after dinner?) And conversely, if all of your coworkers walk together on their lunch break, it's much likelier that you might too.

Increasingly, people are finding that online forums and communities through social media provide a flexible and effective social learning tool, where those with similar challenges and goals and can meet to encourage each other, brainstorm solutions, and report results. Even Stephen Covey, author of the best-selling book *The 7 Habits of Highly Effective People,* has launched an online learning community to create a system for providing support as people work to develop new habits to accomplish shared goals.

There is significant evidence that social support is important in decreasing the effect of chronic diseases and improving overall survival. In fact, one extensive literature review documents consistent evidence linking social support to lower cardiovascular mortality (risk of death due to a cardiovascular cause) and strong evidence that social support predicts survival in cardiac patients.[15]

The same resource shows that research has answered an important question regarding social support: It does predict mortality by any cause. The author contends that social support is not a "magic bullet" against disease, more that it is one of the many pellets that seem to influence mortality. The researchers have compared the strength of social support to the effect of exercise and control of blood pressure. The use of social media and social support for diseases such as back pain have been less studied.

Of course, as we have seen in previous chapters, chronic back pain is an illness with prominent psychosocial components. Our team has noticed that many patients naturally form support groups and thus seem to enjoy better results. Social influences can also have negative effects, however. For example, many patients have been conditioned to believe, and therefore propagate, that all physical therapy is the same or that they need weekly chiropractic adjustments throughout their entire life to prevent pain.

> *Chronic back pain is an illness with*
> *prominent psychosocial components.*

Others believe, based on previous surgical consults or experiences, that there is a surgical solution or quick fix out there for any pain. Some may believe that they are entitled to a pain-free existence without putting in any personal effort. These are each myths that we busted back in Chapter 5. And yet, they remain prevalent because people continue to share them widely and hurt us. So before listening to the mounds of advice from seemingly similar patients, it is important to make sure that you are connecting with like-minded individuals who share similar goals for long-term self-empowerment.

Because it can be hard to find the right people to confide in or take advice from, we actively cultivate the belief and experience that regaining strength and flexibility—and hence improving function—should be the primary goal. Pain will naturally be relieved once strength and flexibility are attained.

Patients are routinely educated about the body's own recuperative capacity and given realistic expectations regarding surgery. We focus patients by helping them realize that success is defined by attaining functional goals, not just by reducing their pain level. We believe that support groups act to quiet those negative voices and inspire patients by highlighting daily and weekly victories.

Three Spine Diagnoses Where Specific Support Groups Are Especially Important

Over time, I have noticed the formation of a few specific informal support groups at SpineZone clinics that have been particularly helpful to their members. One particular support group is made of patients who have had complex spinal disorders like scoliosis or kyphosis. The group is made up of those who are trying to choose the right treatment for relief of their pain, as well as those who have had surgery or have been told by multiple doctors that they definitely needed surgery. These patients have compared and shared success stories of both operative and non-operative treatment with others like them.

The decision to proceed with surgery in this group is a particularly difficult one. Patients must weigh the benefit of surgically straightening their spine with the risks of a multi-level fusion surgery. By fusing the curvature in a better position, patients *can* get pain relief through removal of these unevenly strained disc levels, but what is the right timing for surgery? And further, when can we say that non-operative treatment has "failed"?

It is very important to treat patients with scoliosis and kyphosis in a multi-disciplinary fashion since most trainers and therapists don't have the experience with their difficult deformities. Also, prior to deciding to operate, most surgeons cannot be certain that their patients have received the best therapy for their specific condition, since not all therapy is created equal for every condition. Ideally, any professional guiding the patient will advise them based on a thorough knowledge of the surgery and anticipated post-operative outcome compared to the outcome of the best available non-operative treatment.

Studies show that this extensive deformity surgery has a 50 percent complication rate and a long recuperation period. What's more, it does not guarantee that other disc levels will not become painful and degenerative to require more surgery in the future. As a result, patients faced with the decision to undergo surgery often benefit from the perspective of other patients who have succeeded with and without surgery, and from therapists with experience in this realm. Whatever their decision, these patients need to take deliberate steps to monitor and maintain their back health throughout their lives.

Another support group that seems to naturally form consists of patients who have suffered from disc degeneration, and either had surgery or succeeded through exercise and stretching alone. Patients with significant symptomatic disc injuries or degenerative disc disease, who must either choose fusion surgery or live with their residual back pain, benefit from the perspective of patients who have stayed active years after facing the same decision, through lifestyle and habit changes alone.

This group naturally forms since the surgical solution to back or neck pain due to disc injury or degeneration is fusion, and the success rate of surgery in this population is significantly lower than discectomy surgery for sciatica, for example. Many patients in this group who chose to avoid surgery delight in sharing how well they are functioning despite their condition. This satisfaction continues even over a decade after their decision to commit to an active strengthening and stretching program...one that includes activity modification and postural treatments.

And finally, patients who have had severe sciatica or radiating arm pain due to disc herniation frequently find comfort in each other's stories. They like to share how their symptoms—and even their disk herniation—disappear on the MRI after 6-12 weeks of treatment. Online support groups may offer even more opportunity to better match such patients from a larger pool of those of a similar age, gender, and socioeconomic status.

This group naturally forms since nerve pain due to disc herniation is particularly acute and debilitating. Patients draw from each other's strength and have a better chance of tolerating non-operative treatment. They understand that by waiting 6-12 weeks, by judiciously using medications and injections for only the most severe pain, and by using appropriate targeted stretches and exercises, that they have a high probability of natural resolution of the pain and shrinkage of the disc herniation.

Creating Resiliency Through Social Support Systems

It is well recognized that social support significantly predicts an individual's ability to cope with stress. The fact is, we're just more resilient when we have others we can lean on. Knowing that others value us is an important factor in helping us set aside the negative aspects of our lives so we can focus on thinking more positively about our predicament. It can help prevent anxiety, depression, and even boost our immune system.

Social support significantly predicts an individual's ability to cope with stress.

Interestingly, just as social support keeps us motivated to comply with recommended exercises, exercise can also improve our ability to be social...a sort of virtuous cycle of positive change. This occurs through the production of oxytocin, a hormone we reviewed briefly in Chapter 2. We discussed how women's bodies produce oxytocin, thereby improving pain tolerance in childbirth. But oxytocin does so much more. It even has a role in human social behavior, facilitating the ability to read other people's emotions and deepening bonds between members of a group.

How does this occur? The experience of prairie voles may offer a clue. In one study presented at the Society for Neuroscience in New Orleans, researchers noted that voles that exercised by running on wheels over a period of six weeks showed an increase in oxytocin production.[16] They also bonded rapidly with females in their cages, while the non-exercisers did not.

When it comes to treatment of back pain and the benefits of exercise and social connectivity, these seem to be interrelated. The bottom line here is that to effectively treat chronic back pain, a combination of exercises for strengthening and flexibility are important, as we have discussed. But to make this a habit that sticks, establishing methods to improve accountability can increase the odds.

So don't neglect this aspect of your plan as you begin to put together your own program for a stronger and straighter back. Take a quick inventory: Do you have at least one person in your life who would have the time and interest to serve as your accountability buddy? If not, consider employing the many wearable devices or applications on your phone, or joining a gym or regular exercise program, or engaging in a non-operative treatment program that incorporates the social connectivity of like-minded individuals dealing with similar conditions as yours.

Be Willing to Change, Be Informed… and Be Successful

It's important to realize that many of your daily habits may be working against you and further guiding you toward either surgery or a life of decreased function and persistent pain. When you think about it, this is good news. Knowing what you're doing wrong is the first step to fixing it. You *can* change many of your habits to further your chances for healing and regaining function. Try to use the strategies discussed above to deal with each and every one of these habits in a systematic and patient manner.

If you are facing deformity surgery, make sure that you have received your non-operative treatment from a practitioner experienced in your condition. Also make sure that you have sought out patients facing similar levels of fusion and correction surgery who have been treated both operatively and non-operatively. You want to decide for yourself what is the best outcome you can expect with or without surgery and what complications you may face before you make your decision.

Similarly, if you are facing fusion surgery for disc injury or degeneration, make sure that all other possible sources of pain have been eliminated. Also, make sure that you have been through the best core strengthening program available to strengthen the entire corset of muscles around your spine. I would advise waiting at least six months and preferably greater than one year after the development of severe back or neck pain before undergoing surgery since the odds are that, with strengthening and activity, your pain will subside.

Make sure that this time is spent increasing your activity and strength, improving your posture, and bringing awareness to any underlying anxiety, depression, or catastrophized thinking. Make sure that you have talked to patients who have undergone fusion surgery for similar conditions, not just a few months or years prior, but up to five to ten years after surgery to see what you can expect.

Lastly, if you have arm or leg pain due to a disc herniation, make sure that you have tried the best targeted "centralization" exercises that help decrease nerve irritation and centralize the pain to your back or neck and out of your extremities. Don't rush into such surgery for up to at least six weeks after onset of symptoms if possible, since the odds are on your side to improve without surgery.

If your pain is severe and you don't know if you can tolerate it, recall the many examples of spontaneous relief of symptoms from even large disc herniations. Even though the risk of surgery for this particular condition is low, make sure that you give appropriate consideration to the possible bad outcomes that can arise.

The bottom line with these three scenarios (and essentially with any condition for which you are considering elective surgery) is to adequately assess the risk and benefits in the long-term of surgical treatment compared to the best you can do non-operatively. Don't settle for comparing the outcome of surgery with how you would feel if you did nothing at all to heal your spine naturally. You deserve the best that your body can do on its own before you decide to have surgery. And finally, no matter which treatment you ultimately choose, modify your long-term habits so that you don't suffer from these conditions again.

Key Learning Points: The Impact of Habits

1. It takes time to create habits that are automatic, on average in one study about nine weeks, but the

good news is that interruptions now and then do not affect the habit formation process.

2. There are three phases of habit building: the "honeymoon phase" where you first feel inspired; the "fight-through" phase where you must remain convinced you need to make the change; and the phase where habits become second nature.

3. The scientific literature supports these tips for forming and sustaining a new positive habit: Link the new behavior to a routine, reward yourself, track progress, keep it simple, make a detailed plan, and be accountable.

4. Social support is an important component in acquiring and supporting healthy habits. You can identify an accountability buddy on your own or meet those with similar challenges in selected treatment programs.

CHAPTER 8

DEVELOPING AN EFFECTIVE, INTEGRATED CARE PLAN

"Start by doing what's necessary; then do what's possible; and suddenly you are doing the impossible."

—Francis of Assisi

In the previous chapters, I have outlined many aspects of spine care that I learned out of necessity. While I had acquired this amazing skill to perform spine surgery, I was still faced with the reality that I was only *part* of the solution. As Penney Cowan, founder of the American Chronic Pain Association, has said, "Treating a pain patient can be like fixing a car with four flat tires. You cannot just inflate one tire and expect a good result. You must work on all four."

So I did what was necessary: I opened my eyes to consider all the other factors that affect a good patient outcome—including the series of core-strengthening exercises that our group had designed and perfected over the years. Next, I did what was possible, which was to begin to bring these and other aspects of spine care (such as education, self-empowerment, and psychology) into my practice.

Finally, I acted on my vision, which would have been considered impossible years ago, before healthcare began its shift from a "pay for service" to "pay for performance" model. I brought together multiple—often non-traditional—practitioners with the aim of combining their best practices and cooperating with one another to improve patients' back care. This was how SpineZone was born.

My path and the SpineZone program are in harmony with the evolution of healthcare. Healthcare today is in the midst of seismic change. In fact, a recent article in *Harvard Business Review* opened with the words: "In healthcare, the days of business as usual are over."[1] Everyone who works in healthcare today—physicians, hospital leaders, and insurance companies—understands that high healthcare costs with uneven quality will no longer be tolerated.

In fact, since the implementation of the Affordable Care Act, insurance companies are following the government's lead by rewarding healthcare providers who provide the best outcomes at the lowest cost, rather than basing reimbursement solely on procedures and visits as was done in the past. This model can be good for patients, because increasingly, the patient's best interests are squarely at the center of care...instead of sometimes at the periphery, as we shall discuss further in a moment.

When doctors, hospitals, and insurance companies operate independently, as they have in the past—and still do to some extent—there are conflicting incentives and the patient's needs can get lost in the shuffle. Sad but true.

The Ongoing Quest for Value

In short, providing good *value*—higher quality at a lower cost—is the overarching goal in the new healthcare model. As a result, care is becoming more integrated...which is very good news for those with back pain. As you become better educated about your condition and potential choices for solutions that will meet your goals, it will also become easier over time to identify integrated health programs that provide this type of value.

> *Providing good* value—*higher quality at a lower cost*—*is the overarching goal in the new healthcare model.*

Of course, as a nation we still have a long way to go to achieve these goals. We exist in an imperfect system that is ever evolving. As a spine surgeon, I was trained to work where the "system" was central in healthcare decision making. Under this paradigm (which is still in place to a degree), if you wanted your insurance to cover your condition, you went to your primary care physician, who would help navigate you through the maze of acceptable and covered treatment options such as physical therapy, pain management, or spine surgery.

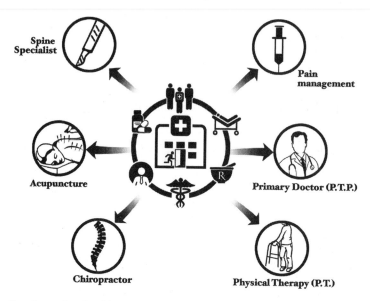

See how the healthcare "system" is decentralized and disjointed. Providers are acting alone, often unaware and uninvolved with what the others are doing. Managing a complex and multi-factorial disease like chronic back pain is made difficult when data and processes are not shared and there is no collective learning. Fortunately, that's changing.

If you didn't like these options, you would have to navigate yourself (sometimes at your own expense) through the maze of possible alternative treatments such as exercise therapy, chiropractic, or acupuncture; needless to say, this could be quite confusing.

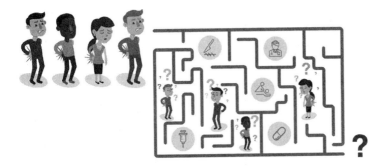

The wide array of choices available for treatment of chronic back and neck pain are difficult to navigate. As a consumer or a healthcare professional, it is difficult to plot a course through this maze to obtain the best value (i.e., high quality care at the lowest possible cost).

I believe that the latest trends in healthcare are aligned with my specific experiences in building SpineZone: The patient is now becoming the *center* of focus. Resources are at the periphery of the patient's needs and are truly delivered in service to the patient's goals, as they should be.

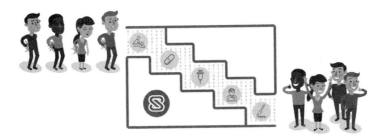

At SpineZone clinics, the patient is now the center of focus. Social, environmental, and behavioral conditions are taken into account throughout the patient's treatment. Resources are tailored to the patient's needs and are truly delivered in service to the patient's goals, as they should be.

Comprehensive, integrated programs like Spine-Zone consider and address the environmental, social, and behavioral needs of patients. Traditional healthcare providers—such as the primary care physician, physical therapist, pain management specialist, and spine surgeon—frequently work together with other allied healthcare providers (e.g., trainers, exercise specialists, mental health practitioners, chiropractors, and acupuncturists) to provide the appropriate level of care to address *all* of the factors that affect the disease we are seeking to treat: chronic back and neck pain, in this case.

> *Comprehensive, integrated programs like SpineZone consider and address the environmental, social, and behavioral needs of patients.*

Hans's Story

One patient who helped me understand the value of an integrated approach to spinal care was Hans, a 67-year-old man who fell off his ladder while putting up Christmas lights one winter. When he began to experience low back pain, he went to see his primary care doctor, who then referred him for six weeks of physical therapy.

After the six weeks, he felt his back pain was better, but still noticed some imbalance when he walked, which was disregarded as a secondary complaint. Three to four weeks later, he returned to see his doctor because he was having some upper back pain (which had been overshadowed due to the lower back pain he experienced as a result of the fall).

Because he'd improved from the first round of physical therapy, he was referred back for his upper back pain and also saw a chiropractor. Yet, his symptoms did not improve. And in fact, he became increasingly unsteady when he walked. Eventually, he came to see me for a surgical consultation.

Past MRI scans of his low and mid back revealed only degenerative disc disease, but his physical examination and persistent difficulty with balance were immediately noteworthy to me. Hans was a very active gentleman who prided himself on his activity and balance, and was frustrated that throughout his treatment, everybody assumed that his lack of balance was because he was old.

When I examined him, I noted that he had abnormal reflexes that pointed me to a problem with his spinal cord that was higher in his spine. After ordering and reviewing new MRI scans of his upper spine and neck, I noticed a large bone tumor that had eroded and weakened the bone resulting in a fracture as a result of the fall. As a result, Hans was developing increasing spinal cord compression that was causing his imbalance.

I do not fault any of the practitioners who treated Hans for not ordering upper spine and neck scans, since they were each focused on his symptoms at the time. He complained about low back pain to his primary care doctor. (On the prescription, the main complaint was written as low back pain, so it is understandable that the recommended treatment concerned only his lumbar spine.)

And then, once Hans reported that physical therapy had helped this problem, his doctors became convinced that he was suffering only from degenerative disc disease or a sprain or strain. So when he then complained of upper back pain, they disregarded it as a significant symptom and elected not to image that area. They also concluded that since he was still able to walk, his balance difficulties were likely longstanding. So they did not concern themselves with it or even address it as a "new" symptom.

The problem was that the early physical therapists and primary care doctors did not share information or perspective about their physical examination findings for Hans with each other. With this lack of integration, it is completely understandable how a diagnosis of such a condition would fall through the cracks. Even in the age of the Affordable Care Act, with its push to share all information electronically, this type of condition would not be caught. This is because the therapist and surgeons often lack direct and frequent communication, let alone co-development of protocols and training to avoid problems such as occurred in Hans's case.

By the time Hans saw me, he was wheelchair-bound and would have likely continued to worsen over time. Without undergoing timely, appropriate surgery to remove the compression on his spine and rid him of the tumor, he would have likely become permanently paraplegic and have prematurely died. This is why integrated care is so important; identifying and communicating issues between different specialists results in better, more coordinated care.

Everybody Wins with Collaboration

Patients benefit enormously when there is a culture of close collaboration between primary care physicians, trainers, physical therapists, pain management specialists, and surgeons. Unique perspectives from care providers with training in different types of disciplines can inform an overall treatment approach, but *only* if everyone is open to feedback and willing to put aside the classically hierarchical Western model of medicine. Exercise physiologists, trainers, and physical therapists have much to teach surgeons about how to effectively treat back pain patients, and vice versa.

> *Patients benefit enormously when there is a culture of close collaboration.*

I first came to understand this when I met George, a well-known 63-year-old ophthalmologist who had struggled for years with back and leg pain. An avid tennis player who was nationally ranked in his age division, he was diagnosed with severe stenosis and spondylolisthesis. By the time we connected, he was resigned to never playing competitive tennis again and was undergoing surgery just to be functional enough to continue work.

He had received multiple opinions from surgeons who all said he would require the surgery, and that his chance of returning to competitive tennis was low. And frankly, the first time I saw him, I agreed. Nonetheless, I referred him to SpineZone to check his muscle strength and ensure that his rehabilitation to date was appropriate.

To my surprise, the rehabilitation team determined that George had significant weakness in lumbar extension, despite the fact that he played tennis (which involves a lot of extension) and worked out in the gym four days a week or more. I had learned in my training that in conditions such as stenosis, patients are more symptomatic when they extend their trunk backwards. As a result, I had cautioned therapists to avoid exercises that involved extension so that they did not reproduce symptoms of pain.

However, the exercise physiologists had noticed this significant deficit in range of motion and strength in extension and recommended that we actually do the opposite of what I suggested...specifically strengthen George's spine in extension. Over time, I've learned that the fact that such patients experience pain upon extension is a clue to their lack of muscle strength, and the key to resolving it is to strengthen these muscles throughout the range of motion of the back.

Once George did this, he returned to playing tennis, and now, four years post-treatment, he is very happy with his long-term results. I credit this success to my astute exercise physiologist who taught me that some of my anatomic and surgical assumptions might not translate to rehabilitation. I also learned how even classic surgical conditions—those where I would have predicted a need for surgery to correct—are actually well treated with the appropriate focused exercise and strengthening.

And last, I learned how much of a dramatic impact a sustained strengthening and conditioning program could have on an appropriately motivated patient. Even though George was better after 10 weeks of treatment, it took him five months to obtain above normal strength throughout his range of motion and be able to play tennis painlessly. Without a sustained program that provided progressive strengthening in a medical setting (where the complexity of his condition was well understood), he would not have been able to obtain this excellent result.

Integrated Care Is Gaining Traction in the Treatment of Common Conditions

The value of this type of integrated team approach has already become increasingly common in other medical specialties. In cardiac programs, for example, there is feedback and cooperation between the cardiologist, cardiothoracic surgeon, and cardiac rehabilitation physicians.

In diabetes, there are multi-disciplinary teams that include an endocrinologist who has expertise in the disease and understands how to manage the ramifications of the hormone imbalance and changes in blood sugar levels. This team also includes sub-specialists—like ophthalmologists and nephrologists—who can manage the visual and kidney problems that arise in diabetics.

It's important to recognize that no one specialist in medicine is best qualified to manage all aspects of a certain disease. Many factors contribute to making a person sick and it is difficult and perhaps impossible for one specialist to "go at it alone" in launching a treatment plan that will work for the patient. This is the power of a multi-disciplinary approach. In breast cancer, oncologists and surgeons team with psychologists to provide a holistic approach to managing the many psychological, physical, and emotional aspects of breast cancer. *All areas of the healthcare industry should be making strides such as these.*

> *Recognize that no one specialist in medicine is best qualified to manage all aspects of a certain disease.*

We Need to Go Further to Best Treat Back Pain

When it comes to treating back pain, there have been multiple attempts at integrating care. There have been many experiments to better integrate spine care. One of them is the advent of functional restoration programs. This workers' compensation program lasts six weeks and integrates physical therapy, psychological treatments, and pain management. While I have seen some good results and many studies have shown these programs to be effective, I find that the help they offer patients is often too little, too late, and at too high a cost.

One problem is that these multi-disciplinary spine programs have often been reserved until close to the end of a patient's treatment, once he has already been labeled as a "failed back patient" or become chronically addicted to increasing doses of narcotic pain medication. They are usually not integrated with a surgeon, so the messaging is often inconsistent. And though these programs provide six weeks of intensive treatment and are definitely at least partially successful, they are also very expensive for the workers' compensation insurance system. To provide some context, these six-week programs cost about $40,000, while SpineZone's ten-week programs—which admittedly require patients to be onsite for fewer hours at a time—cost a small fraction of this.

I have seen many of these patients revert to their prior state after completing the six-week program. It's easy to see why. Frankly, it seems unlikely that many years of habits would be reversed with a six-week program that fails to provide additional long-term support if a patient "falls off the wagon." Therefore, in my opinion, such programs do not provide a sustainable long-term solution to the chronic back patient's problems.

In my experience, the process of integration is most effective when it begins early in the patient's journey and addresses as many of the sub-specialties that need to be involved in the care of their disease. It must also achieve excellent outcomes in the most cost-effective way.

Virginia Mason's Model for Spine Care

One such example of spinal care is a program at Virginia Mason Medical Center in Seattle. At Virginia Mason, physical therapists work closely with the physical medicine and rehabilitation physicians. Patients are frequently seen by each of these team members on the same day and then begin therapy.

By integrating the physical therapist and rehabilitation physician teams, they've been able to design a coordinated program that results in fewer missed work-days for patients and that requires fewer physical therapy visits. They even reduced the use of MRIs by 23 percent while improving outcomes.[2] (However, physical therapists and rehabilitation physicians are not the only kinds of practitioners who can treat spinal conditions. Just imagine the potential positive impact for patients if a much larger cross-section of diverse practitioners were all working together in this same way!)

One characteristic that many successful multi-disciplinary groups share is that, in addition to providing treatment, they also assume responsibility for engaging the patient and families in the care they provide. This involves counseling, encouraging prevention, and supporting new healthy behaviors, like smoking cessation or weight loss.

On this type of team, everyone knows and trusts one another, which frequently improves both communication and clinical results. Teams are also incentivized toward the success of the *patient* rather than the success of any specific sub-specialty or individual practitioner.

In other words, in the example of Virginia Mason, even though the physical therapists may see the patients much less frequently than they otherwise might, they are incentivized to meet overall patient improvement goals so the interests of the patient take priority over their own self-interests.

What makes the most difference for patients in an integrated care unit is not fancy job titles or even physically locating the staff together, but rather, consistent opportunities to collaborate on treatment and review the data on how the group is performing. They must take full responsibility as a team for improving the full cycle of care.

> *What makes the most difference for patients is collaborating on treatment and consistently reviewing the data on how the group is performing.*

The SpineZone Approach

SpineZone offers an additional example of how integrated care can work to help patients with back pain recover. By considering the approach we use, you can gain a sense of what components you may want to seek out in an integrated program for your own recovery.

It begins with screening. Our solution to integrate back care efficiently at SpineZone begins with a screening process to identify patients with possible "red flags" that might indicate they are not a good fit for non-operative care. For example, there are warning signals in the patient's history and exam that can signal a more severe underlying condition, such as an infection or cancer. If these warning signs are identified, further examination or diagnostic studies such as X-rays or MRI scans are recommended and ordered.

The screening process also identifies "yellow flags," which are signals that pose possible pitfalls in non-operative care. (Some patients have undergone multiple previous surgeries or are overly focused on an MRI abnormality, for example.) These patients will likely benefit from more explanation from either the spine surgeon or the physician assistant who works with them to put concerns to rest and feel confident in a positive outcome without surgery.

> *The screening process also identifies "yellow flags," which are signals that pose possible pitfalls in non-operative care.*

Often when a patient isn't confident about non-operative treatment—when they are instead focused on quick fixes or surgical treatments (as we have seen in the examples of some patient stories in previous chapters)—this approach is doomed from the outset. That's why patients appreciate our integrated approach since a spine surgeon or specialized physician's assistant can address their specific surgical concerns.

They understand that specialty care is not being withheld from them. A spine surgeon is actively involved in diagnosing their condition, reviewing any available imaging studies, and monitoring progress to recovery. Importantly, since the team meets weekly for training webinars and in person monthly, the ongoing training and cross-education of the staff allows the trainer to be able to speak in general terms about surgery, and the surgeon to more adequately address rehabilitation.

Also, by sharing examples of other patients with similar conditions who recovered successfully without an operation (and explaining proactively how many people have MRI abnormalities without pain), patients feel empowered and stay committed to a prolonged program of targeted strengthening and postural treatment.

An exercise physiologist is key. The next ingredient for success is focused strengthening with an exercise physiologist or certified trainer who specifically understands spine conditions and the specialized techniques that are necessary to rehabilitate the spine as compared to the extremities. When a professional athlete sustains an injury and needs to return to function, to whom do they turn? They frequently enlist the aid of the team trainer or exercise physiologist. Even though we have fewer demands on our bodies than professional athletes do, why should we settle for treatment that's less effective? Doesn't the quality of everyone's life and earning potential depend in large part on their function?

An exercise physiologist (or kinesiologist) has earned a bachelor's degree (or sometimes a more advanced degree) with coursework in biology, anatomy, chemistry, and physiology. This specialty is concerned with the analysis, improvement, and maintenance of health and fitness.

And increasingly, exercise physiologists are recognized as vital members of the allied health professions, for rehabilitation of chronic diseases like heart disease and disabilities caused by conditions of the spine, for example. An exercise physiologist has specific expertise and training to condition a person to a higher level of fitness and health, while maintaining awareness of safety issues like underlying diseases or illnesses and minimizing the risk of injury or environmental exposure.

While you may be familiar with exercise physiologists who work in non-clinical settings like health clubs or with athletic teams, *clinical* exercise physiologists are trained to offer medically supervised exercise programs. The most common of these types of programs treat patients with heart and lung disease and cancer. Medically supervised exercise programs for weight loss and programs for senior citizens are also well recognized.

Exercise physiologists are particularly well suited to treating chronic spine conditions due to their focus on function. In our SpineZone clinics, they are well versed in spinal conditions since they undergo regular training and education sessions as an integrated group. They also have easy access to both the spine surgeon and physician assistants for specific questions that arise with patients.

They employ the best available training methods for the core spinal muscles with a focus on measuring strength and then comparing it to the strength of similar patients without back or neck pain. They then empower patients to sequentially improve strength to match or surpass expected normal strength levels.

Addressing the psychological component is important. Just as there are many types of practitioners who can help patients regain strength, so too are there many types of mental health practitioners—psychologists, psychiatrists, marriage and family therapists (MFTs), and licensed clinical social workers (LCSWs)—who are well qualified to address the psychosocial issues that are so commonly experienced with spinal conditions.

However, the beauty of SpineZone's integrated approach is that members of the interdisciplinary team are trained to look for and address any misperceptions about disability or feelings of disempowerment early.

We bust those myths before they become more intractable challenges that can be managed only through a more time-intensive, costly process with specialized psychological or psychiatric therapists.

> *Members of the interdisciplinary team are trained to look for and address any misperceptions about disability or feelings of disempowerment early.*

In most cases without underlying significant diagnosed psychological abnormalities, there's no need for specific psychological counseling because the clinical team can act together to build and support a patient's confidence in a non-surgical solution. By discussing their examination findings and diagnostic studies, the team (which includes the exercise physiologist, physical therapist, physician assistant, and surgeon) can credibly address patients' areas of concern together.

By educating the patient on areas where their fears do not match reality, they can avoid the psychological downward spiral that can ensue for some patients when they feel pain and worry about long-term outcomes. The minority of patients who have severe anxiety or depressive conditions can then be specifically referred to mental health professionals.

We know that lasting change takes time. A *sustained* program is necessary to both strengthen effectively and also for an exercise physiologist to build sufficient rapport to relieve the anxiety and depression that sometimes come with back pain. (I am convinced that one of the reasons we have been so successful at SpineZone is that one of our earliest partners, Sharp

Community Medical Group in San Diego, agreed with us that the sustainability of the program was one of many keys to its success. They allowed their patients up to 20 visits upon initial referral without any need to return back for reauthorization. In our current disjointed health system, where often only four to six visits of physical therapy are authorized at a time, this was a big step.)

We monitor posture. Since maintaining good posture is so important in everyday life, one of the components of SpineZone is a postural monitoring system where we take pictures at regular intervals and evaluate postural abnormalities that often can be overlooked. By helping patients develop self-awareness of these abnormalities, we have been able to significantly improve their postural habits. Unless there is a concern about scoliosis or another significant structural issue, I find X-rays to be unnecessary during routine postural analysis.

> *SpineZone uses a postural monitoring system where we take pictures at regular intervals and evaluate postural abnormalities.*

We know that certain conditions are particularly responsive to specialized rehabilitation techniques. For example, there are decades of research on a technique called the McKenzie Method for treatment of specific types of disc herniation. Success has also been documented with certain treatments for scoliosis. Since SpineZone is an integrated program that is based on the best scientific evidence available, we are actively engaged in using research across disciplines in our treatment approaches.

We address pain (most often without medication). Not all patients progress easily through rehabilitation. Sometimes individuals with severe nerve irritation from the disc and resultant severe leg pain (sciatica) cannot perform the exercises they need to do to get stronger. Other patients may experience severe pain when they bend backwards or twist. This occurs when the facet joint (the small joint in the back that we discussed earlier) becomes irritated. In such cases, these patients may require an injection near the disc or in the facet joint to relieve some of the irritation and inflammation so that they can resume their rehabilitation activities.

This is another benefit of an integrated program like SpineZone. We can identify these conditions quickly to provide the appropriate level of care so the patient isn't bounced back and forth between different groups and specialists.

In fact, we find that primary care doctors also prefer our integrated treatment model because they can confidently refer a patient to one place without the need to choose between physical therapy, pain management, chiropractic care, or surgery. In my experience, they appreciate being part of the integrated spine team, because patients with back conditions typically need a lot of time and education on these complex conditions and they understand that we are well equipped to provide it.

Best of all, we can usually help patients minimize or even eliminate their pain without prescribing potentially addictive opioid medications. Often patients are able to stop or at least reduce usage of previously prescribed drugs. In fact, in a sample of 121 of our patients who completed the program since August 1, 2015, there was an overall 74 percent reduction in use of medications between their initial visit and their final visit. We saw a 67 percent reduction in narcotics, a 75 percent reduction in anti-inflammatories, and an 81 percent reduction in muscle relaxants. The message is clear: When you provide another way to address pain, patients just don't need the pills.

We monitor progress closely. To ensure we are always achieving results in the most efficient way possible, we developed a sophisticated computer program to monitor patient progress. First, we collect data on patients' personal characteristics and condition. Then we track their improvements in strength and function.

> *First, we collect data on patients' personal characteristics and condition. Then we track their improvements in strength and function.*

With this data, we have also been able to improve our treatment protocols. For example, we noticed that patients who had greater than two previous attempts at non-operative treatment were not completing the program at the same rate as others. By addressing their pessimism early, we increased their compliance in the program significantly. And over time, our compliance rates continue to increase.

As we continue to collect more data, we hope to be able to predict the outcome of specific patient populations. For example, if we know that diabetic men between the ages of 30 and 45 with disc herniations take over 30 visits to obtain the strength gains necessary to improve their function, we can set appropriate expectations for those patients from the onset and ensure we provide an adequate level of resources. These types of statistics are particularly valuable to physicians as we attempt to predict required resources to achieve desirable outcomes in the industry's shift towards population health.

Embrace Your Body's Ability to Heal

Perhaps the most important ingredient for a successful and effective recovery from back pain is a patient's own belief in the power of his or her body's recuperative ability. My father taught me that through his own example.

At 78, he sustained what is called a "flipped bucket-handle tear" of the meniscus in his knee. In other words, the cushion in his knee tore and became trapped in the knee joint so that he could not fully extend his knee. (There was also a large fragment of cartilage that was rubbing against the surface of his knee.)

My brothers—who are also orthopedic surgeons—and I sent him to an orthopedic colleague who diagnosed the problem and recommended surgery. (In fact, there isn't a single surgeon in the country who would have advised my father to skip surgery. His injury was severe.)

So you can imagine the shock and dismay of my brothers and me—three surgeons—when he announced his intention to repair his injury through rehabilitation. When we expressed our concern about his knee becoming permanently bent, he asked, "What if I work really hard to get it straight again?" We were skeptical, but he was resolved. He refused to have the surgery.

He asked what he needed to do to optimize his results, so we taught him some exercises. But we also made him agree that if he couldn't fully extend his knee in four weeks that he would undergo surgery. Otherwise, we were afraid his knee would be stuck in a bent position. Not only would he be unable to play tennis, but he would also likely limp and have significant challenges walking.

For more than six hours per day over the next four weeks, my dad was rigorous about adhering to his stretching routine. And you know what? He regained his full range of motion. Not only did he succeed in avoiding surgery, but he was back on the court playing tennis within two months!

To this day, he continues to garden and remain quite active. After his success, my brothers and I reviewed some older cases in the literature and found that some patients had in fact resumed nearly normal athletic activities with injuries like his. While we had reflexively recommended surgery due to our training, he taught us to embrace the profound healing potential that is possible without surgery…to truly consider each patient's individual condition and be open to a wide range of options for rehabilitation.

My father is another surprising example of just what a highly motivated person can accomplish when he wishes to avoid surgery. And today, I can point to many, many examples of patients with severe pain or injury who have healed just as profoundly. My greatest wish is for you too to experience dramatic pain relief and recovery to reclaim a joyful and active life. If my dad can do it, so can you.

Navigating Healthcare Today: How You Can Stay at the Center of the System

Remember that as our healthcare system evolves and continues to improve, it is your job to ensure that *you* remain at the center of your wellness experience. This will probably require you to take a more proactive approach than you are used to, but the result will be that you are able to guide your journey back to health. This means that you will be less likely to fall into the "system"—a slippery slope that many times leads to unnecessary injections or surgery. Below you will find lots of great questions to ask your physicians and surgeons along your path to recovery.

Initial Questions to Ask Your Doctor After a Spinal or Neck Injury

You have just injured your back and limped in to see your primary care doctor. Here are some essential questions to ask at this appointment:
- What do you think is causing my pain/disability?
- What is the average recovery time for this type of back/neck injury?
- When is the earliest I can return to stretching, walking, stationary bike, treadmill, or gym activities?

- If you are sending me to physical therapy, how well do you know them and how specialized are they at treating spinal conditions?
- What should I be doing outside of physical therapy to help me heal and prevent this from happening again?
- Do I have any "red flags" that may warrant further investigation?
- If you want me to have an injection, what are the risks and benefits of this? Other than temporary relief, is there any long-term benefit with the injection?
- Do you think I have a good understanding of my condition? If not, what resources are available?
- If you are sending me for an injection or a surgical consultation, can I come back and talk to you about what they say to see what you would do in my position?
- What is the gentlest pain management treatment option for this type of injury?

Questions to Ask Your Surgeon/Physician When Surgery Is Not Mandatory (Elective) or When You Suspect It Is Too Soon for Surgery

Now that you have read this book, you understand that doctors sometimes turn to surgery as a premature "last resort." Armed with this knowledge, you will be better equipped to question your need for surgery after an unsuccessful round of physical therapy or a few injections that haven't quite done the trick. Here are some questions to prompt a dialogue if you hope to avoid surgery and want to allow your back to heal naturally:

- What would happen to my condition if I didn't have this procedure?
- Have you seen cases like mine in which the patient was able to tolerate their symptoms without undergoing surgery?
- What is the harm in delaying this procedure for six months or a year?
- Can I wait a few weeks and come back to see whether my condition has worsened or improved?
- What can I do to prevent this from happening again?
- What lifestyle changes do I need to make?
- If you or a family member were in my position, would you undergo this procedure?
- Is this the least invasive way to treat my condition?
- What are the consequences to the rest of my spine (the muscles and the other discs) if I undergo this procedure?
- Do you feel that I have done all that I can do non-operatively? If not, are there any other options that have a chance to help me avoid surgery?
- If I undergo this surgery, what are the chances that I will be able to keep running/gardening/picking up my toddler (insert your functional goal)? This is part of my lifestyle and is extremely valuable to me, and I want to return to it soon.
- What would happen if I modified my activities and elected not to pursue some of them? Could I then prevent the need for this surgery?

Questions to Ask Your Doctor as You Continue on Your (Surgery-Free) Path to Recovery

Congratulations! You have decided to safely pursue a natural solution to your back pain. Remember, this is a marathon—not a race. As you move forward with your team of experts, be sure to keep the dialogue going so you continue receiving the best treatment options for your particular condition.

- How often should I follow up with you to gauge my progress?
- Should I try acupuncture/personal training/meditation/other alternative therapy as a mode of maintenance moving forward?
- What diet/lifestyle changes should I engage in to rid my body of excess inflammation?
- What is my ideal weight for my height/gender and how can I achieve or maintain it?
- How can I best build and maintain core muscle strength?
- What can I do to improve my posture so I avoid as much deterioration as possible?
- Can you recommend an integrated ongoing treatment program to help me pursue my healing naturally and safely?

Ultimately, you are your own best advocate. It is my belief that most physicians and other healthcare professionals care deeply about their patients. However, they cannot help but view you through the lens of their training and the environment they practice in daily. Only you can decide whether you are willing to accept the risks of surgery vs. the responsibility of a more natural approach to healing your back (or any other part of your body for that matter).

My advice is simple: Learn everything you can about your back and how it works. Do everything possible to follow the advice in this book and to live a healthful lifestyle in general. Talk over all of this thoroughly with your physician. Finally, think long and hard before you make a decision to undergo elective surgery. There *are* risks with any surgery, and you should weigh these risks against your most probable benefits from the intervention.

Sometimes surgery is the best decision. Sometimes it's not. But in the end, if you make the effort to take charge of your health, you will be able to look back with no regrets and with the realization that you did the best you could with the knowledge you had—and that peace of mind is incredibly valuable.

Key Learning Points: Developing an Effective, Integrated Care Plan

1. Providing good *value*—higher quality at a lower cost—is the overarching goal in the new healthcare model. As a result, care is becoming more integrated, with the patient and their needs at the center of focus...which is very good news for those with back pain.
2. Motivation and a willingness to commit to beneficial stretches and strengthening exercises are often the main factors that determine whether or not a person will experience natural healing of their back

condition. Many psychological barriers to improvement are removed with appropriate medical exercise treatment. Even people in their 70s, 80s, and 90s can heal and regain mobility with enough determination.

3. You can and should fully participate during your doctor appointments. While a physician can help you unlock your healing potential and give you the tools to succeed, your input and engagement are vital. By coming to your appointments already educated about your condition and prepared to ask and answer questions about your unique circumstances, you can help take charge of your healthcare experience.

4. Typical multi-disciplinary spine treatment programs can be expensive and ineffective for patients with chronic back pain, unless they allow for long-term access and follow-up. They are often reserved for "failed back patients" and those addicted to pain pills. Further, these programs, which often last only six weeks, do not go far enough with treatments, and, unfortunately, often set the patient up to revert back to old, destructive habits.

5. Patients benefit greatly from a culture of collaboration. They ultimately have better outcomes when primary care physicians, trainers, physical therapists, pain management specialists, and surgeons are able to work together to create a cohesive treatment plan. Seek out these types of collaborative systems for the most well-coordinated care. SpineZone has been designed specifically to put patients at the center of the healthcare system—right where they belong.

CHAPTER 9

BEST PRACTICES FOR A HEALTHY SPINE

Hopefully, this book has helped you learn some valuable truths about your back or neck pain. I have tried to paint a picture of the importance of muscle strength and posture, but also of releasing unhealthy thoughts and maintaining a positive perspective as you go about your life. Unfortunately, when all doesn't go well, injury or discomfort and pain often result. I hope you now see that your back and neck pain do not exist in a vacuum—on the contrary, many powerful factors determine how you experience pain and whether your muscles are healthy and strong or weak and ineffective at stabilizing your joints.

Not all surgery is unnecessary, and there are readers who may most definitely need to have it. I have reviewed those instances in previous chapters.

However, I believe that surgery is rarely the best answer to treating most cases of back and neck pain. I have seen too many people heal on their own—even those with significant MRI abnormalities—without needing to go under the knife. I've also seen too many surgery patients face complications or endure lengthy recuperation periods, at times without the long-term results that they expected.

My team at SpineZone has worked to find solutions that empower patients like you to continue living their lives while strengthening their spine in a guided and supportive environment. I hope that you will empower yourself by maximizing core strength, idealizing body weight and diet, and educating yourself about your condition before undergoing any elective spine procedure.

After reading this book, I hope you have a new sense of optimism about combating your back condition by unbridling your body's healing potential. Maybe your surgeon has advised you to hold off on a procedure since the benefits don't clearly outweigh the risks. Or perhaps your primary care physician wants to "wait and see" if the tenderness in your low back continues before making a referral or ordering an MRI. Maybe you've undergone a few weeks of physical therapy but still have lingering discomfort. In those cases, where surgery isn't the obvious course of action, what can you do to improve your chances of finding natural relief?

I believe the path to pain relief and increased physical and emotional strength lies in the way you treat your body, mind, and soul. In the following pages I have listed some practical steps you can start taking today in order to start seeing results tomorrow. (Most of them are covered in more detail throughout my book.) These are the best practices that you can engage in to maintain your healthy back—or to get back the health that you lost.

Tackle Obesity and Weight Management

If you are overweight and suffering from back pain, you owe it to yourself to do a reality check. Chances are, the extra pounds you are carrying take a daily toll on your quality of life. I have repeatedly seen the effects obesity has on my patients' spines and on their lives in general. Though I am not a nutrition specialist, I have been amazed by how following a few simple rules can make such a dramatic difference in patients' health. In fact, I have often been told by overweight patients who have lost weight that they no longer wish to proceed with surgery.

I urge you today to do some research on how to safely lose weight. Either ask your primary care physician for information or consult a nutritionist to find a system that works for you. Many people find success by cutting down on carbohydrates, while others embrace a vegan or vegetarian lifestyle. Still others find that keeping their diet basically the same but counting calories and practicing portion control is an effective approach to weight loss.

Portion control is key in any diet, but it's important not to "starve" the body. You have to remember, the human body has adapted for survival, and food was not always abundant. When your body enters into this "Starvation Mode," due to a lack of adequate nutrition, it slows down its metabolism and more calories are stored as fat, to be used only out of absolute necessity.

It's essentially a preparatory step your body takes to ensure survival.

This is why it is important to spread out your intake so that you eat six meals a day of varying sizes. When you do this, your body sees that there is adequate nutrition in your immediate environment and that there is really no need to store it as fat for later emergency use. Also, try to give your bowels a break by leaving 10-12 hours after the last meal of the day before you eat again in the morning.

Exercise, of course, is almost always helpful for weight loss. While I do believe the foods we choose are the most important factor—I've seen estimates that weight loss is 75 percent diet and 25 percent exercise—regular cardio and muscle building efforts are also vitally important. Regular exercise and maintaining adequate lean muscle mass are key to increasing your metabolism, so you can lose weight all day long. It's just hard to lose weight while living a sedentary life—and moving your body is important for many other reasons as well.

Keep in mind that the food and exercise tips listed in this chapter (and explained in detail throughout this book) can also help you lose weight. You will find that as those extra pounds come off, you will feel more in control, more energetic, and ready to work on healing your spine.

First, know your BMI. A good guideline to help you determine your ideal weight is the body mass index (BMI), which can easily be calculated by knowing your height and weight and using online tools. Check your BMI now to help gauge how much weight you may need to lose. Ideally, a BMI of less than 25 is considered healthy. (It's also important to know that BMI may overestimate body fat in athletes and others who have a muscular build, and conversely it may underestimate body fat in older persons and others who have lost muscle.)

Cut out the excess sugar—especially processed sugar. This means cutting out most desserts, sodas, sugar-laden junk foods, and fruit juices (yes, juice is loaded with sugar!). The most appropriate time to include simple sugars that you would get from fruit is earlier in the day, or either before or after your workout. Oatmeal and mixed berries would be an example of a good source of energy and antioxidants prior to a workout, while a banana could be great after a workout.

Control carbs by "carb cycling." Carbohydrates themselves are not the villain; it's the type of carbs and the times they are ingested that can either do harm or good. Carbs are actually very important for building muscle, losing weight, and maintaining an overall healthy and active lifestyle. You can think of carbs as the "energy workers" that take the bricks, or proteins, and build the foundations for healthy muscle.

First, you should try to eat only complex carbs such as whole grain bread, beans, potatoes, oatmeal, or brown rice. It's best to avoid (or at least minimize) simple carbs such as white bread, pasta, and sugary foods or desserts. Then practice carb cycling, which means letting your activity levels dictate your carb intake.

Try to eat your carbs early in the day and at the post-workout meal. Do not eat carbs too close to bedtime since your activity level and expenditure of energy are decreased (I recommend stopping carbs at 6:00 p.m.). On your most active days or days where you are strengthening your legs and back, ingest complex carbs to a maximum of 1 to 1.5 grams per pound of body weight (usually around 200 grams). All other gym days (or moderately active days) would be medium carb days; strive for around 150 grams. All non-gym or inactive days should be low carb days (around 100 grams).

When trying to severely reduce the amount of carbs, choose healthy fats such as mixed nuts, extra virgin olive oil, fatty fishes, avocados, ground chia seeds, and minimal amounts of cheeses. Most of these ingredients would work really well in a leafy green salad that could pair well with any lean protein. The result is a filling and satisfying evening meal that satisfies all the key nutritional points.

Ditch the "diet" anything! Diet foods, in particular, are full of chemicals that want to trick your brain into feeling satisfied. They are addictive and are often loaded with sugar and salt to compensate for being low fat or fat free. These synthetic foods are best avoided and should be replaced with natural food.

Don't eat deep fried foods. Most commercial deep fried foods are prepared in dangerous, hydrogenated oils that quickly go rancid and can destroy your health over time. In general, it is better to eat raw and/or fresh foods or ones that have been cooked at lower temperatures over a longer time, rather than foods that have been cooked quickly at very high temperatures.

Choose fresh over processed. If it comes wrapped in plastic, chances are that it is processed (think cookies, chips, breakfast cereal, etc). Get rid of these processed foods and replace them with healthy whole foods instead.

Read your food labels. It is important to know what you *are* eating when you tear into a package of food. Reading your labels gives you an idea of the quality of food products and can alert you to the presence of unsavory additives and preservatives. Remember, if you can't pronounce it, you probably shouldn't be eating it anyway. Get to know the ingredients in your foods and become aware of those you should and should not be eating. Essentially, the longer the ingredients list on an item, the more processed and inherently worse it is for you.

Be active each day. It is a good idea to be physically active every day as you try to lose weight. If you are used to being sedentary, start walking 30 minutes a day two times a week for the first week. Then work up to 30 minutes a day five times a week. You will likely need to push yourself beyond some self-imposed limits, but make sure your physician clears you for exercise first. Remember that small increments of effort pay off over time. Take it slow and steady until you are ready to increase your intensity levels.

Weight training and muscle building. Increasing muscle mass increases your metabolic rate, which means that you will burn more calories all day, even when you are not exercising. It is important to add this element to your regimen two times a week. Building muscle requires that you exercise it to its limit to break it down, then allow that muscle to rebuild itself with rest and proper nutrition. Be sure to eat some protein after each weight training session. (See Chapter 6 for more details.)

Monitor your progress in inches, not pounds. Generally, it is a good idea to pay attention to inches lost instead of pounds lost. Your weight can fluctuate close to 10 pounds daily due to water intake, food, clothes, and excretion. Remember that muscle weighs more than fat, so even as you lose fat, the scales could still stay the same. While you don't really need to weigh yourself each week, consider measuring your belly and monitoring your weight loss through inches lost from your stomach each month. I'd also recommend taking this a step further and keeping a photo log. It is easy to take photos with your phone weekly or monthly to track progress. You will be delighted to see your progress play out in this manner.

Pace yourself. When you are trying to lose weight, don't be a weekend warrior (someone who trains hard only a few days a week and is otherwise sedentary). This is a good way to injure your spine and other joints—especially if you are new to exercise. Space your workouts so that you are getting regular exercise and not overexerting yourself to the point of injury.

Fuel Your Body with Spine-Friendly Foods (and Plenty of Water Too!)

All food, even the "junk" variety, keeps us alive. But food should do more than just sustain us. If you eat the proper diet, your food will not only give you daily energy, but will also nourish your body and help it perform better. Back health and good nutrition go hand in hand. Hydration also plays a vital role, as your back needs lubrication in order to function at its best. Follow the tips below to ensure that you give your body the fuel it needs to thrive and support a healthy spine:

Get an appropriate amount of protein. Make sure you are ingesting about 25 to 30 grams of protein per meal—any more than that will likely be turned to fat if you don't use it as energy. That's the amount found in four ounces of lean meat or a three-egg-and-cheese omelet. This amount will maximally stimulate muscle build-up when and if you work out. Also, try to ingest some protein within 30 minutes after resistance training to build up muscle.

Enjoy as many vegetables as you want. In addition to getting ample protein, you should feel free to eat as many vegetables as you want. Vegetables are nutrient dense and provide the body with health-generating vitamins and minerals. In addition to eating an array of vegetables each day, add a green salad to *any* meal to help fill you up and fuel you on your journey toward better health.

Focus on inflammation-fighting foods. A major factor that contributes to back and neck pain is the presence of inflammation in the joints and tissues of the spine. You can help control inflammation through the foods you eat. In addition to choosing whole, real foods, you should reach for choices that are naturally anti-inflammatory: high-fiber veggies, colorful fruits, salmon, olive oil, legumes, nuts, alliums like onions and garlic, and even the occasional glass of red wine. You can find a more detailed list of inflammation-fighting foods in Chapter 2.

Drink water, lots of it. Proper hydration helps the spine by lubricating your discs and keeping you limber. To make sure you're getting enough fluids, sip water throughout the day—it's the very best liquid you could choose to drink. Keep a bottle of water on your desk and be sure to take a drink every few minutes. If plain water gets boring, keep things interesting by adding orange, lemon, or cucumber slices. Or try carbonated water for some fizz (but only occasionally since too much carbonation has its down sides).

As you take steps to hydrate, it's still important to reduce or eliminate your caffeine intake. Caffeinated drinks like soda and coffee actually contribute to dehydration. Substitute caffeine-free herbal tea for a calming alternative.

Minimize your alcohol intake. Alcohol is a diuretic, meaning that it causes you to pass more urine. When it enters the system, the body immediately attempts to flush out the harmful substance by releasing water from water-storing cells. This is what leads to dehydration, hangovers, and upset stomachs.

Not only does alcohol decrease hydration, but it is also a depressant that can be addictive. I have seen many patients who self-medicate with alcohol. It contributes to a cycle of decreased motivation, sleep disruptions, weight gain, and a general lack of self-control. While the occasional glass of wine is fine, you should generally keep your drinking to a minimum.

Heal Your Spine Through Exercise

It can be tricky to navigate the world of exercise when you are recovering from a spinal injury. But it is also important to support your body through an appropriate level of physical activity, dictated by the circumstances of your condition. If you have been inactive up to this point, know that a fitness routine will improve many areas of your life—not just your spine health. Speak with your doctor about how you can safely stay (or become) active and strong as you recover. Below are several tips and tools you can incorporate into your fitness routine:

Get a great gadget. Use a Fitbit, Jawbone, Apple watch, or similar device to measure your daily activity level. Aim for getting 10,000 steps in each day to combat weight-related back pain.

Find apps you love. Applications such as Nike Training Club or the activity application on iPhones are good ways to log and track your exercises. There are also many nutrition tracker apps that can help you keep a handle on your food choices.

Schedule your exercise. Pencil in your workouts on a calendar so you are more likely to do them! This helps you view your workouts as a previous commitment and keeps you accountable. Workout journals where you list what you did and when are great for accountability too.

Warm up before lifting. It's vitally important to warm up prior to doing a strenuous activity. Before you lift anything (be it a weight at the gym or an everyday item like a sack of potatoes), warm up by lifting something less heavy first. Pre-loading the disc at a lower resistance decreases the risk of injury to the disc and prepares it for bearing a larger load.

Stabilize your spine. Do the spine stabilization exercises as described in Chapter 6 at least five times a week. These exercises strengthen the transversus abdominis (TA) and the multifidus. They are the muscles that embrace and support the spine, so it's to your benefit to work on them regularly.

Do a "doorway" stretch for relief. A simple door-frame can help you stretch out your upper back and shoulder muscles any time you need it. Place your hands on the sides of a doorframe as you advance through the threshold. This allows you to stretch your chest and shoulders in one easy movement. Do this each time you approach a doorway.

Periodically stretch to rehydrate your discs. During prolonged times of exercise or other vigorous activity (such as yard work), lie down for five minutes and do some stretching, including a full forward bend to help rehydrate your discs. Do this every two hours, especially if you are doing continuous or repetitive bending or lifting.

Make the most of gym equipment. In the gym, use the Roman chair (see Chapter 6) to gain strength through the entire range of motion. This exercise is done face down and allows you to do a "reverse sit-up" by bracing you behind your ankles and in front of your abdomen. This is a great exercise you can do during your workouts to start combating weakness.

Have a ball. An exercise ball (also called a "Swiss ball" or "physio ball") is an inexpensive device you can use for simple home exercises like sit-ups. (As a bonus, you can also use this as a chair at your desk. Replace your normal chair with the ball for 30 minutes a day to help engage your core.)

Approach HIIT (high intensity interval training) workouts with caution. If you choose to participate in high intensity strength training programs, such as CrossFit, Insanity, or P90X, don't sacrifice on form. It is much better to do fewer reps and maintain healthy spine posture throughout than to risk injury that comes from poor form and pushing through exhaustion.

Remember the importance of social support. Exercise is much easier when you have a buddy to inspire you and help keep you accountable! You and a friend can schedule walks or sweat sessions at the gym together.

Take your dog for a walk or a run. Not only is this a great way to work out, but the bonding you and your dog experience will keep the happiness factor strong (and experiencing joy daily is an important component of wellness that will positively affect all areas of your life).

Consider practicing yoga or Pilates. Both yoga and Pilates can provide beneficial strengthening and stretching for the spine. A beginning level of yoga is often gentle enough to accommodate people who have been sedentary for years. Make sure not to force yourself into the postures.

Cat-cow is one of the simplest stretches you can practice, but it provides big relief after a tense day. Practice it frequently to ease tired or tense back muscles. See Chapter 5 for a detailed description of this stretch.

Build conditioning into your day. Pull in your stomach muscles when you bend over to tie your shoes or pick up your child. Take the stairs anytime you see them. Do stretches during commercial breaks. There are endless ways to improve your health in tiny increments that won't feel overwhelming.

Take "back" breaks during exercise. Vigorous exercise requires that you take breaks to ease the tension in the back muscles. This will also help "rehydrate" your discs. Your spine will thank you (and that goes for totally healthy spines as well!). For example, if you are a long distance runner, be sure to take a break at least every hour to rehydrate the disc and help avoid injury.

Daily Habits to Embrace

Over time, the daily choices you make *become* your life habits. This is why every health-based decision you make is so important. If you spend years stooped over a desk while eating a poor diet and avoiding exercise, you may be putting yourself at risk for disc damage and back pain in the future. Here are a few great habits to start hardwiring now:

Do vital exercises at the same time daily. Certain beneficial exercises (for example, activating the TA muscles) should become habitual. When you establish an official time to perform these exercises (like first thing in the morning, or just after dinner), you reinforce the habit so it becomes second nature.

Create cues for healthy habits. Remember the "doorway" stretch? The reason this stretch is so great is because over time, the simple act of approaching any doorway will serve as a "cue" to remind patients suffering from neck and back pain or tightness to stretch and then reset their posture. Do this each time you approach a doorway and it will soon be automatic. Also consider using a Fitbit as a cue to be more active. It is hard to miss that bright band on your wrist, and it's a constant reminder that you need to be hitting 10,000 steps.

Practice sitting correctly. Any time you sit in a chair (for example, when working at a desk, eating a meal, or even driving) avoid the C shaped posture that can be damaging to your spine and muscles. Follow the detailed instructions found in Chapter 2 on how to sit properly.

Set reminders to adjust your posture. As you are getting used to practicing better posture, set a timer to go off every 30 minutes to remind yourself to check on your spine positioning, along with your neck, head, and shoulders to ensure that you are properly supporting your frame.

Take breaks from sitting every 30 minutes. At the very least be sure to stand up and move around every hour. Go for a short walk (even if it is just down the hall!) and consider doing some light stretching, just to ensure that your blood is flowing.

You can also try out a standing desk. Or if you are so inclined, spend some time sitting at a regular desk and then move over to work at a standing desk or at a counter top. Make sure to elevate your computer monitor to eye level so you don't have to bend your neck or lean down to see the screen.

Be aware of your posture when you are driving. Follow the detailed instructions from Chapter 2 to learn how to lengthen your spine and "lock" your elongated posture onto the back of your car seat.

Use posture apps. If you want to work more on improving your posture, there's a great app for that. Check out the PostureScreen app to help monitor your posture and see how it improves over time. Also consider wearables such as Lumo Lift, which remind you to adjust your posture whenever you slouch.

If you carry a purse, wear it across your body. Many people carry purses and satchels over one shoulder, but this strains your spine and nervous system. Instead, wearing it cross body helps distribute the weight and keeps your body in alignment.

Keep your wallet slender and in your front pocket. Don't carry around credit cards you don't need all the time. The thinner your wallet, the less your body has to compensate for the uneven strain it causes. And whenever possible, store your wallet somewhere other than your back pocket.

Carry your backpack on *both* shoulders. Encourage your kids to do the same so they start developing healthy habits today. This is particularly important that kids do this, as their spines are still developing.

Avoid "text neck." Remember that certain repetitive movements can cause damage over time. Looking down while texting is a prime example of improper bending. When you pick up your smartphone to send a text, hold it higher and look down with your eyes to avoid bending your neck.

Plan ahead so you'll actually implement healthy habits. Pack your gym bag the night before you plan to work out. Prep veggies ahead of time so you can cook healthy meals minus the stress. It is helpful to use a whiteboard in a bedroom or chalkboard in the kitchen to schedule weekly meals, log diets, and plan workouts. Thinking one step ahead sets you up for success and helps reinforce healthy habits.

To reinforce your good habits, find ways to reward yourself. For example, if you enjoy television, then let yourself relax and watch a show. But on the commercial breaks, do some of the home conditioning stretches found in this book. This way, a potentially burdensome task (stretching or doing stabilization exercises) has a reward (television) built right in.

Center yourself daily. Every day, it is very important to find a few quiet moments to become present and experience peace. When you are dealing with an injury of any kind, it is just as important to work on your inner state as it is to tend to your physical well-being. Set aside time each day for meditation or a simple deep-breathing practice.

Make joy a habit. It is incredibly important to seek out joy every day. Joy is good for your soul and can be a powerful motivating factor in healing your spine. Be sure to laugh with your friends and family often. Watch a funny show on television. Spend time with loving pets. Read more about healthy habits in the next section: "Attitude Adjustments."

Attitude Adjustments

I have explained how important it is to avoid catastrophic negative thinking. I can't reemphasize it enough: Your outlook will profoundly affect your entire healing journey. It is imperative that you acknowledge your feelings of hopelessness and sorrow and gradually replace them with the positive response your body experiences after exercise and activity. It is also important to know that your wellness is always in flux and to remind yourself that your point of view can either help or hurt your prognosis. I encourage you to embrace hope and be willing to try instead of giving up. Here are several tips to help you take an optimistic proactive role in your recovery:

Live in the present. I can't emphasize this enough. If we all truly lived only in the present most of the time, many of our problems would cease to be seen as problems. I recommend *The Power of Now* by Eckhart Tolle for detailed instructions on how to stay in the present.

Embrace daily positive habits. Try meditation or self-guided relaxation exercises. Better yet, do a meditation retreat or attend group meditation. Be sure to find a way to tune in to yourself every day. If you begin a meditation practice (and I strongly encourage you to be open to it), you will come to enjoy this special time in which you get to connect your consciousness with your subconscious. Plus, meditation truly makes you feel better thanks to its calming effect. I like the "Breathe" app, which provides many different, intention-specific, guided meditations.

Take stock of your negativity. Many people are shocked when they realize how often they think negative thoughts. Keep a notepad with you for a day and add a tick mark each time you catch yourself thinking a negative thought. This awareness will help you realize how much power your negative thoughts really possess.

Now, consciously replace those negative thoughts with positive ones. This can be very difficult to do when you are in pain, but I promise they will make your pain more bearable over the long haul. You can't change the condition you are in right now, but you can change how you approach your injury.

Take a 10-second mental break any time. Any time you are feeling discouraged or upset due to your pain or injury (or for any reason, really!), give yourself permission to take a mini break.

Stop everything. Breathe for a few quiet seconds. Let everything that is bothering you fall away. It really works, so use this tactic often to keep your general outlook positive and hopeful.

Know that your spine is much more than your MRI results. If you are focused on your MRI or X-ray findings, read about and learn how many normal people with absolutely no pain have significantly abnormal findings.

Use your affirmations to remind you that you *can* heal! It's too easy to get discouraged when you're in pain, but the truth is, a negative mindset will hold you back from healing. Refer often to the affirmations I have included in Chapter 4. You can even write your own. Repeat them daily and remind yourself that with each new day you are one step closer to healing.

Rely on friends and family for support. Your loved ones can have a grounding effect on you during times when your pain tries to "take over" your life. Have a few trusted companions on speed dial who agree to lend you support any time you need it. Call them up if you need a shoulder to lean on, when you need fresh perspective, or when you need to stop the cycle of catastrophic negative thinking.

Pain Management

As we discussed earlier, opioids are overprescribed, addictive, and dangerous. In an effort to lessen the stronghold that opioids have held over the healthcare industry, doctors are beginning to focus on non-narcotic solutions for ongoing pain management.

Luckily, certain low-risk standbys are still effective today, minus the risks associated with pain pills. These techniques may help you out when you are in discomfort:

Start with initial rest. In general, inactivity is not advised, but in a state of acute severe pain, a period of rest for 24 to a maximum of 48 hours can help calm the pain enough. Then start with gentle stretches and gradually increase your activity level as you continue to heal.

Soothe the injury with heat/ice therapy. Generally, it's best to use cold therapy—either with ice packs or even a frozen bag of peas—when there is a more acute injury. Apply a cold pack in increments consisting of 20 minutes on, then 20 minutes off. It is important not to apply either cold or heat therapy directly to your skin. Use a thin buffer, like a hand towel. Heat is generally helpful for more chronic pain or a spasm. In those cases, I specifically like ThermaCare heatwraps. They provide long-lasting, low-level heat for the back or neck.

Try over-the-counter pain medications. Tylenol is a good pain reliever, but it is important not to take too much (less than 4,000 mg/day). Tylenol can be taken in conjunction with anti-inflammatories. I find ibuprofen (Motrin) to be very helpful. You can take up to 800 mg, three times a day, but make sure that you don't have any abdominal discomfort and avoid ibuprofen if you have a history of ulcers. Naproxen (375 mg), taken twice a day is an alternative if ibuprofen doesn't work.

Use pain relief gels. There are many over-the-counter pain relief gels that work well to treat discomfort. If your pain is more severe, Voltaren Gel can help, but it requires a prescription. (Don't use a heating pad after you have applied a topical product because that combination can increase your risk of burns.)

Do a trial of traction. Traction stretches the back or neck to take pressure off of discs. The traction can be applied either manually or with a mechanical traction device. You can ask your physical therapist to try manual traction. (As far as mechanical devices go, I find the Saunders unit to be useful for patients with severe neck pain or arm pain due to disc herniations.) For treating the low back, I often recommend using an inversion table, which is similar in effectiveness to more expensive spinal decompression therapy. While it does work to increase the space available for the nerves and may help the disc get more nutrition, the effects of traction are neutralized as soon as you go back to standing against gravity. I should also state here that there is no evidence that traction provides long-term benefits.

Try meditation or guided imagery. I have found the focus and self-realization brought about by even simple meditation techniques to be very helpful for pain relief and also for calming anxiety. Don't underestimate the power of the mind-body connection. See Chapter 3 for detailed instructions on the basics of meditation. Also, try the Breathe application for some simple guided meditations.

Feel electrified with TENS. Transcutaneous electrical nerve stimulation (TENS) is the use of electric current produced by a device to stimulate the nerves for treatment of either acute or chronic pain. Those who use it wear a battery-powered device with electrodes placed on the skin over the painful area. The TENS unit then blocks pain signals through electrical impulses, which changes the perception of pain. While early studies seemed to show that TENS increased endorphins, more recent studies have had mixed results on its effectiveness in treating low back pain.

Explore biofeedback. Biofeedback is commonly used for back pain. Electrodes are attached to the skin, which then relay information about breathing, muscle tension, heart rate, and skin temperature to the electromyography machine. The patients then learn how to regulate their response to pain by practicing relaxation techniques that affect these bodily processes. However, there is not yet much real evidence that biofeedback has a clear benefit for low back pain.

See if acupuncture or massage works for you. Acupuncture can help lessen pain (it's been found to be moderately useful for low back pain) and also helps wean patients off of pain medications. It's even effective at treating anxiety and depression. The theory is that by inserting small needles into certain points in the body, practitioners can clear blockages in Qi, which the Chinese recognize to be the "life force" of the body. An explanation more in line with Western medicine might be that these needles stimulate chemicals within the body—such as endorphins and serotonin—that are released. In any case, many clinical studies continue to investigate the value of acupuncture, with conflicting results to date.

Also, for symptomatic relief of pain—especially if you have spasms—try massage. You can either visit a massage therapist or explore self-massage techniques. Many people swear by massage (at the very least, it can be a relaxing way to spend an hour).

Visit your doctor for prescription-strength medication or injections. There are many options for prescription medication. Topical medication, like Voltaren Gel mentioned above, or Lidoderm (pain relieving) or Flector (anti-inflammatory) patches, can provide local relief from pain. There are also stronger and different types of anti-inflammatory medication protocols, including a short course of steroids, which can be very helpful. Muscle relaxant medications can help with spasms. Narcotic pain medications are useful for severe, unremitting pain, but avoid asking for courses of narcotic pain medications that last more than three to five days.

Know that epidurals offer temporary relief. Epidurals are a short-term fix for pain. They only decrease inflammation around the nerve and do not treat the underlying process. Like medication, traction, manipulation, and TENS, epidurals are very useful during the acute phase of an injury and should be used accordingly. It's important to recognize they do not represent a long-term solution to back pain.

No matter where you're starting from right now, know that you can claim control over your health. Let go of negative mindsets and have faith that your body is capable of natural healing. After that, it's all about making the best choices for you and your spine. Those choices will lead you to hope, empowerment, and strength. A healthy and happy spine is waiting for you. Take it back.

RESOURCES

Recommended Books:

Back in Control: A Spine Surgeon's Roadmap out of Chronic Pain by David Hanscom, MD

Back Sense: A Revolutionary Approach to Halting the Cycle of Chronic Back Pain by Ronald D. Siegel, PsyD; Michael H. Urdang; and Douglas R. Johnson, MD

The Body Fat Breakthrough: Tap the Muscle-Building Power of Negative Training and Lose Up to 30 Pounds in 30 Days by Ellington Darden, PhD

8 Steps to a Pain-Free Back by Esther Gokhale, LAc

Healing Back Pain: The Mind-Body Connection by John E. Sarno, MD

If You Like Exercise...Chances Are You're Doing It Wrong: Proper Strength Training for Maximum Results by Gary Bannister, BA, BPE, MEd

In Arthur's Shadow—Daily Musings on Exercise: A Tribute to Nautilus Inventor Arthur Jones by Gary Bannister, BA, BPE, MEd

Movement, Stability & Lumbopelvic Pain: Integration of Research and Therapy, 2nd Edition by Andry Vleeming, PhD, PT; Vert Mooney, MD; and Rob Stoeckart, PhD

The New High Intensity Training: The Best Muscle-Building System You've Never Tried by Ellington Darden, PhD

The Pain Survival Guide: How to Reclaim Your Life by Dennis C. Turk, PhD; and Frits Winter, PhD

Persuasive Technology: Using Computers to Change What We Think and Do (Interactive Technologies) by B.J. Fogg

The Power of Now: A Guide to Spiritual Enlightenment by Eckhart Tolle

Three-Dimensional Treatment for Scoliosis: A Physiotherapeutic Method for Deformities of the Spine by Christa Lehnert-Schroth, PT

Treat Your Own Back, 9th Edition by Robin A. McKenzie

Treat Your Own Neck, 5th Edition by Robin A. McKenzie

The Unguarded Moment: A Surgeon's Discovery of the Barriers to Prescription of Inexpensive, Effective Healthcare in the Form of Therapeutic Exercise by Vert Mooney, MD

The Untethered Soul: The Journey Beyond Yourself by Michael A. Singer

Recommended Websites:

www.takebackcontrol.com
Please visit the website based on this book to explore some back strengthening exercises that you can do at home and other helpful resources.

www.spinezone.com
This is the website for Dr. Raiszadeh's medical clinic for non-surgical treatment for back and neck pain. Please view the video on the home page regarding the back muscles. Also visit the educational section for short videos on different spine-related topics.

www.arthritis.org
Plenty of good advice on proper diet and exercise for arthritic conditions.

www.gokhalemethod.com
Visit this site for reinforcement of proper sitting posture.

www.arthurjonesexercise.com
Arthur Jones was a pioneer of high intensity training and inventor of Nautilus exercise equipment.

www.behaviormodel.org
A great site to explore to understand what triggers behavioral change.

www.dhamma.org
Visit for more information on Vipassana meditation and courses.

www.mindfulness-solution.com
A great source for mindfulness meditations.

www.orthoinfo.aaos.org/menus/spine.cfm
The American Academy of Orthopaedic Surgeons' patient information site for spine issues and treatments.

GLOSSARY

Adjacent Disc Disease—A condition where discs that border a spinal fusion surgery degenerate prematurely.

Ankylosing Spondylitis—An inflammatory disease that can cause vertebrae to fuse together, making the spine rigid and often bent in a hunched-forward posture.

Anterior Cruciate Ligament (ACL)—One of the four knee ligaments that connect the tibia and femur. This ligament stabilizes the knee when the foot is planted and when changing direction.

Apex—The point of the most curvature in the spine.

Biofeedback—A pain relief treatment that involves electrodes attached to the skin. Information about breathing, muscle tension, heart rate, and skin temperature is relayed to the patient in order to learn how to modulate response to pain through relaxation techniques.

Cerebral Spinal Fluid (CSF)—A clear, colorless body fluid bathing the brain and spinal cord.

Cervical Spine—The section of the spine located at the neck.

Cognitive Behavioral Therapy (CBT)—A therapeutic approach for effectively treating chronic pain where the individual learns to recognize negative thoughts and feelings that occur due to back pain and change them into healthy thoughts and actions.

Dark Disc—A term used to describe the nucleus of a dehydrated or degenerated spinal disc that's seen as dark on a certain MRI sequence called T2-weighted. The normal nucleus of the disc is bright on this MRI sequence. Dark discs are not necessarily an indicator that spine surgery is needed or in fact that anything is "wrong."

Degenerative Disc Disease—Describes the changes that occur in the disc as we age. This occurs in everybody, so this is not a "disease" per se, no more than other signs of aging like wrinkles or grey hair. In a minority of cases, symptoms of pain (and sometimes radiating weakness or numbness) can come from a degenerated disc in the spine.

Decompression—A term that's most commonly used when referring to a surgical procedure aimed at decreasing pain due to pressure on a pinched nerve. It is also used to describe the surgery to treat stenosis or disc herniation. Finally "spinal decompression" is used to describe a type of traction therapy used to relieve pain caused by herniated or bulging discs.

Disc Herniation—A condition describing the circumstance when the outer layer of a disc tears, such that the inner layer protrudes. The protruding portion of the disc can press on or irritate the nerves. Many disc herniations can reabsorb on their own without surgery for an excellent long-term outcome. Herniated discs may be classified as protruded, extruded, or sequestered. The type of herniation is not as important as the symptoms that it causes. Many disc herniations are found incidentally in patients who have never experienced pain.

Dura—Membrane that surrounds the sac of nerves in the lower back and seals the spinal fluid that bathes the brain and spinal cord. A tear in the dura due to surgery can result in leaking of spinal fluid, severe headaches, and infection.

Epidural—The space just outside the dura (the membrane that surrounds the spinal cord and spinal fluid). Medication is delivered here through a catheter.

Exercise Physiologist—An individual with specialized training for medically supervised exercise programs.

Facet Joints—Small joints in the spine that enable flexibility for bending and twisting. Healthy facet joints have cartilage that allows the vertebrae to move smoothly against each other without grinding.

Fusion—The process of permanently connecting two or more vertebrae, usually with surgery. The techniques of fusion are designed to mimic the normal healing of broken bones.

Hypertrophy—A term that literally means enlargement. When used in the context of activity or exercise, hypertrophy is the process whereby muscles break down and then rebuild to become larger and stronger.

Hyperlordosis—A condition that occurs when the lower back arches excessively, often resulting in increased joint and muscle stress to the point of muscle pain or spasms. Excessive lordosis is commonly called "sway back," "hollow back," or "saddle back."

Lamina—The back part of vertebra that covers your spinal canal.

Laminectomy—The removal of the lamina to enlarge the spinal canal to relieve pressure on the spinal cord or nerves. Also known as decompression surgery.

Lordosis—The normal sway or inward curvature of the lumbar and cervical regions of the spine.

Lumbar Spine—The section of the spine in the lower back.

Kyphosis—Excessive "roundness" of the spine, also known as "round back" or "hunchback."

Osteonecrosis—A loss of blood flow to bones resulting in death of bone tissue.

Multifidus—A short but stout muscle deep in the spine that works to stabilize the joints and therefore protect them from undue stress. This is the key stabilizing muscle of the spine and the one that is most frequently weak when we develop back symptoms.

Pedicles—Bony structures that connect the vertebral body to the lamina (broad flat plates of bone behind the spinal canal). The pedicles and lamina form a hollow archway to protect the spinal cord and nerves.

Proprioception—Refers to sense of position. It is our ability to know where our body is positioned in space.

Sacroiliac (SI) Joint—Joint below the low back between the sacrum (triangular bone) and ilium of the pelvis, which are joined by strong ligaments. It can sometimes cause pain that is confused with pain coming from the spine.

Scoliosis—A spinal disorder where there is an abnormal lateral curvature and rotation of the spine (often C-shaped or S-shaped).

Somatization Disorder—Characterizes significant complaints about bodily pain and other physical problems that cannot be fully explained by a medical condition. This often occurs when a person feels extreme anxiety about physical symptoms such as pain or fatigue.

Spondylolisthesis—A condition in which one of the bones of the spine (vertebra) slips in relation to the vertebra below it. At times this can cause pain and nerve compression. This condition can be present without causing any symptoms.

Stenosis—The narrowing of the spinal canal, which can cause pressure on the spinal cord and nerves.

Lumbar stenosis occurs in the lower back and can result in limitations in walking and pain in the buttocks or legs. Cervical stenosis occurs in the neck and can result in neck or arm pain, weakness, or imbalance.

Tension Myositis Syndrome—Pain that results from deep, unresolved emotional issues that manifest as chronic back, neck, and limb pain, as well as gastrointestinal and dermatological issues and even repetitive strain injuries. Term coined by John E. Sarno, MD.

Thoracic Spine—The mid-region of the spine. This section normally has a C-shaped curve.

Transcutaneous Electrical Nerve Stimulation (TENS)—A battery-powered device that is worn with electrodes that send small electrical currents to the area of pain. These currents are used to block the pain signal.

Vertebral Artery—Major arteries in the neck that pass through a small tunnel in the bone to supply blood to the brain.

REFERENCES

INTRODUCTION

1. Manchikranti, L. 2000. "Epidemiology of low back pain." *Pain Physician* 3 (2): 167-192.

2. Ibid.

3. 2004. "Lost-Worktime Injuries and Illnesses: Characteristics and Resulting Days Away from Work, 2002." *Bureau of Labor Statistics.* http://www.bls.gov/news.release/archives/osh2_09252004.pdf.

4. "New York State Workers' Compensation Board Return to Work Program." *Workers' Compensation Board.* http://www.wcb.ny.gov/content/main/ReturnToWork /RTW_Handbook.pdf.

5. Luo, X., R. Pietrobon, S. X. Sun, G. G. Liu, and L. Hey. 2004. "Estimates and patterns of direct health care expenditures among individuals with back pain in the United States." *Spine (Phila Pa 1976)* 29 (1):79-86.

6. 2014. United States Bone and Joint Initiative: The Burden of Musculoskeletal Diseases in the United States (BMUS). Rosemont, IL.

7. Ibid.

8. Ibid.

9. 2011. Relieving Pain in America: A Blueprint for Transforming Prevention, Care, Education, and Research. Washington, DC: Institute of Medicine.

10. Ibid.

11. "National Institute on Drug Abuse (NIDA)." National Institute on Drug Abuse. http://www.drugabuse.gov/.

12. Fox, M. 2015. "CDC Finds 'Alarming' Increase in Drug Overdoses." *NBC News.* http://www.nbcnews.com/health/health-news/drug-overdose-deaths-hit-new-record-u-s-cdc-says-n482746.

13. Dowell, D., T. Haegerich, and R. Chou. 2016. "CDC Guideline for Prescribing Opioids for Chronic Pain." *Centers for Disease Control and Prevention.* http://www.cdc.gov/mmwr/volumes/65/rr/rr6501e1.htm.

CHAPTER 1

1. Davis, J. 2009. "Strong Quadriceps Protect Women's Knees from Pain." *Arthritis Foundation.* http://www.arthritistoday.org/news/women-quadriceps-knees.php.

2. LaBella, C. R., W. Hennrikus, and T. E. Hewett. Council on Sports Medicine and Fitness, and Section on Orthopaedics. 2014. "Anterior cruciate ligament

injuries: diagnosis, treatment, and prevention." Pediatrics 133 (5):e1437-50.

CHAPTER 2

1. LaBella, C. R., W. Hennrikus, and T. E. Hewett, e1437-50.

2. Battie, M. C., T. Videman, L. E. Gibbons, L. D. Fisher, H. Manninen, and K. Gill. 1995. "1995 Volvo Award in clinical sciences. Determinants of lumbar disc degeneration. A study relating lifetime exposures and magnetic resonance imaging findings in identical twins." *Spine (Phila Pa 1976)* 20 (24):2601-12.

3. Battie, M. C., T. Videman, E. Levalahti, K. Gill, and J. Kaprio. 2008. "Genetic and environmental effects on disc degeneration by phenotype and spinal level: a multivariate twin study." *Spine (Phila Pa 1976)* 33 (25):2801-8.

4. Solovieva, S., J. Lohiniva, P. Leino-Arjas, R. Raininko, K. Luoma, L. Ala-Kokko, and H. Riihimaki. 2002. "COL9A3 gene polymorphism and obesity in intervertebral disc degeneration of the lumbar spine: evidence of gene-environment interaction." *Spine (Phila Pa 1976)* 27 (23):2691-6.

5. Friberg, S., and C. Hirsch. 1992. "Anatomical and clinical studies on lumbar disc degeneration. 1950." *Clin Orthop Relat Res* (279):3-7.

6. Riseborough, E. J., and R. Wynne-Davies. 1973. "A genetic survey of idiopathic scoliosis in Boston, Massachusetts." *J Bone Joint Surg Am* 55 (5):974-82.

7. Ward, K., J. Ogilvie, V. Argyle, L. Nelson, M. Meade, J. Braun, and R. Chettier. 2010. "Polygenic inheritance of adolescent idiopathic scoliosis: a study of extended families in Utah." *Am J Med Genet A* 152A (5):1178-88.

8. Levine, James A. *Get Up!: Why Your Chair Is Killing You and What You Can Do About It.* New York: St. Martin's Griffin, 2014, 21.

9. Gokhale, Ester. *8 Steps to a Pain-Free Back.* Oregon, IL: Quality Books, Inc., 2008, 38-51.

10. Ibid.

11. Sugiyama D., K. Nishimura, K. Tamaki, G. Tsuji, T. Nakazawa, A. Morinobu, S. Kumagai. 2010. "Impact of smoking as a risk factor for developing rheumatoid arthritis: a meta-analysis of observational studies." *Ann Rheum Dis* 69 (1):70-81.

12. Sköldstam, L., L. Hagfors, and G. Johansson. 2003. "An experimental study of a Mediterranean diet intervention for patients with rheumatoid arthritis." *Ann Rheum Dis* 62:208-214.

13. Parksinson, L., and R. Keast. 2014. "Oleocanthal, a Phenolic Derived from Virgin Olive Oil: A Review

of the Beneficial Effects on Inflammatory Disease." *Int J Mol Sci.* 15 (7): 12323–34.

14. Nenonen, M.T.,T.A. Helve,A.L. Rauma, and O.O Hän-ninen. 1998."Uncooked, lactobacilli-rich, vegan food and rheumatoid arthritis." *Br J Rheumatol* 37:274-281.

15. Min, S.Y., M. Yan, S.B. Kim, S. Ravikumar, S. R. Kwon, K. Vanarsa, H. Y. Kim, L. S. Davis, and C. Mohan. 2015. "Green Tea Epigallocatechin-3-Gallate Suppresses Autoimmune Arthritis Through Indoleamine-2,3-Dioxygenase Expressing Dendritic Cells and the Nuclear Factor, Erythroid 2-Like 2 Antioxidant Pathway." *J Inflamm (Lond)* 12:53.

16. Ma, Y., J. A. Griffith, L. Chasan-Taber, B.C. Olendzki, E. Jackon, E.J. Stanek III, W. Li, S.L. Pagato, A. R. Hafner, and I. S. Ockene. 2006."Association between dietary fiber and serum C-reactive protein." *Am J Clin Nutr.* 83 (4): 760–766.

17. Clinton, C. M., S. O'Brien, J. Law, C. M. Renier, and M. R. Wendt. 2015. "Whole-Foods, Plant-Based Diet Alleviates the Symptoms of Osteoarthritis." *Arthritis* Volume 2015, Article ID 708152, 9 pages.

18. Coghill, R. C. 2010."Individual differences in the subjective experience of pain: new insights into mechanisms and models." *Headache* 50 (9):1531-5.

19. Ibid.

20. Koyama, T., J. G. McHaffie, P. J. Laurienti, and R. C. Coghill. 2005. "The subjective experience of pain: where expectations become reality." *Proc Natl Acad Sci U S A* 102 (36):12950-5.

21. Eippert, F., J. Finsterbusch, U. Bingel, and C. Buchel. 2009. "Direct evidence for spinal cord involvement in placebo analgesia." *Science* 326 (5951):404.

22. Kiecolt-Glaser, J. K., T. J. Loving, J. R. Stowell, W. B. Malarkey, S. Lemeshow, S. L. Dickinson, and R. Glaser. 2005. "Hostile marital interactions, proinflammatory cytokine production, and wound healing." *Arch Gen Psychiatry* 62 (12):1377-84.

23. Wang, Y. L., Y. Yuan, J. Yang, C. H. Wang, Y. J. Pan, L. Lu, Y. Q. Wu, D. X. Wang, L. X. Lv, R. R. Li, L. Xue, X. H. Wang, J. W. Bi, X. F. Liu, Y. N. Qian, Z. K. Deng, Z. J. Zhang, X. H. Zhai, X. J. Zhou, G. L. Wang, J. X. Zhai, and W. Y. Liu. 2013. "The interaction between the oxytocin and pain modulation in headache patients." *Neuropeptides* 47 (2):93-7.

24. Landgraf, R., R. Hacker, and H. Buhl. 1982. "Plasma vasopressin and oxytocin in response to exercise and during a day-night cycle in man." *Endokrinologie* 79 (2):281-91.

25. Hill, E. E., E. Zack, C. Battaglini, M. Viru, A. Viru, and A. C. Hackney. 2008. "Exercise and circulating cortisol levels: the intensity threshold effect." *J Endocrinol Invest* 31 (7):587-91.

26. Jones, M. D., J. Booth, J. L. Taylor, and B. K. Barry. 2014. "Aerobic training increases pain tolerance in healthy individuals." *Med Sci Sports Exerc* 46 (8):1640-7.

27. Harber, V.J., and J.R. Sutton. 1984. "Endorphins and Exercise." *Sports Med* 1 (2):154-71.

28. Melone, Linda. "4 Big Benefits From Strength Training." Arthritis Foundation, Accessed November 27, 2014. http://www.arthritistoday.org/about-arthritis/types-of-arthritis/rheumatoid-arthritis/daily-life/staying-active/strength-training-benefits.php.

29. Jansen, I., D. S. Shepard, P. T. Katzmarzyk, and R. Roubenoff. 2004. "The healthcare costs of sarcopenia in the United States." *Journal of the American Geriatric Society* 52:80-5.

30. Ibid.

31. Ibid.

32. Nelson, M. E., M. A. Fiatarone, C. M. Morganti, I. Trice, R. A. Greenberg, and W. J. Evans. 1994. "Effects of High-Intensity Strength Training on Multiple Risk Factors for Osteoporotic Fractures. A Randomized Controlled Trial." *Jama* 272 (24):1909-14.

33. Paddon-Jones, D., and B. B. Rasmussen. 2009. "Dietary protein recommendations and the prevention of sarcopenia: protein, amino acid metabolism and therapy." *Curr Opin Clin Nutr Metab Care* 12 (1): 86-90.

34. Ibid.

35. Symons, T. B., M. Sheffield-Moore, R. R. Wolfe, and D. Paddon-Jones. 2009. "A moderate serving of high-quality protein maximally stimulates skeletal muscle protein synthesis in young and elderly subjects." *J Am Diet Assoc.* 109 (9):1582-6.

36. Schumann, J. H. "If Slow is Good for Food, Why Not Medicine?" *NPR.* http://www.npr.org/blogs/health/2014/12/05/368736643/if-slow-is-good-for-food-why-not-medicine.

CHAPTER 3

1. Kanaan, R.A.,T. K. Craig, S. C.Wessely, and A. S. David. 2007. "Imaging repressed memories in motor conversion disorder." *Psychosom Med* 69 (2):202-5.

2. Carson, A. J., B. Ringbauer, J. Stone, L. McKenzie, C. Warlow, and M. Sharpe. 2000. "Do medically unexplained symptoms matter? A prospective cohort study of 300 new referrals to neurology outpatient clinics." *J Neurol Neurosurg Psychiatry* 68 (2):207-10.

3. Nimnuan, C., M. Hotopf, and S. Wessely. 2001. "Medically unexplained symptoms: an epidemiological study in seven specialities." *J Psychosom Res* 51 (1):361-7.

4. Snijders, T. J., F. E. de Leeuw, U. M. Klumpers, L. J. Kappelle, and J. van Gijn. 2004. "Prevalence and predictors of unexplained neurological symptoms in an academic neurology outpatient clinic–an observational study." *J Neurol* 251 (1):66-71.

5. Schechter, D., A. P. Smith, J. Beck, J. Roach, R. Karim, and S. Azen. 2007. "Outcomes of a mind-body treatment program for chronic back pain with no distinct structural pathology–a case series of patients diagnosed and treated as tension myositis syndrome." *Altern Ther Health Med* 13 (5):26-35.

6. Rhudy, J. L., and M. W. Meagher. 2000. "Fear and anxiety: divergent effects on human pain thresholds." *Pain* 84 (1):65-75.

7. Portenoy, R. K., and K. M. Foley. 1986. "Chronic use of opioid analgesics in non-malignant pain: report of 38 cases." *Pain* 25 (2):171-86.

8. Linnman, C., L. Becerra, and D. Borsook. 2013. "Inflaming the brain: CRPS a model disease to understand neuroimmune interactions in chronic pain." *J Neuroimmune Pharmacol* 8 (3):547-63.

9. Gruson, K. I., K. Huang, T. Wanich, and A. A. Depalma. 2013. "Workers' compensation and outcomes of upper extremity surgery." *J Am Acad Orthop Surg* 21 (2):67-77.

10. Board, New York State Workers' Compensation. 2014. "Return to Work Program." New York State

Workers' Compensation Board Accessed December 19, 2014. http://www.wcb.ny.gov/content/main/ReturnToWork/ReturnToWork.jsp.

CHAPTER 4

1. Zigler, J. E., R. W. Warren, and D. D. Ohnmeiss. 2016. "Comparison of 1-Level Versus 2-Level Anterior Cervical Discectomy and Fusion: Clinical and Radiographic Follow-Up at 60 Months." *Spine* 41 (6):463-9.

2. Fountas, K. N., E. Z. Kapsalaki, L. G. Nikolakkakos, H. F. Smisson, K. W. Johnston, A. A. Grigorian, G. P. Less, and J. S. Robinson Jr. 2007. "Anterior cervical discectomy and fusion associated complications." *Spine (Phila Pa 1976)* 1;32 (21):2310-7.

3. Hilibrand, A. S., G. D. Carlson, M. A. Palumbo, P. K. Jones, and H. H. Bohlman. 1999. "Radiculopathy and myelopathy at segments adjacent to the site of a previous anterior cervical arthrodesis." *J Bone Joint Surg Am* 81 (4):519–28.

4. Mochida, K., H. Komori, A. Okawa, T. Muneta, H. Haro, and K. Shinomiya. 1998. "Regression of cervical disc herniation observed on magnetic resonance images." *Spine (Phila Pa 1976)* 23 (9):990-5; discussion 996-7.

5. Benson, R. T., S. P. Tavares, S. C. Robertson, R. Sharp, and R. W. Marshall. 2010. "Conservatively treated

massive prolapsed discs: a 7-year follow-up." *Ann R Coll Surg Engl* 92 (2):147-53.

6. Gatchel, R. J., and K. H. Rollings. 2008. "Evidence-informed management of chronic low back pain with cognitive behavioral therapy." *Spine J* 8 (1):40-4.

7. Smeets, R. J., J. W. Vlaeyen, A. Hidding, A. D. Kester, G. J. van der Heijden, and J. A. Knottnerus. 2008. "Chronic low back pain: physical training, graded activity with problem solving training, or both? The one-year post-treatment results of a randomized controlled trial." *Pain* 134 (3):263-76.

8. Gatchel and Rollings, 40-4.

9. Hauner, K. K., S. Mineka, J. L. Voss, and K. A. Paller. 2012. "Exposure therapy triggers lasting reorganization of neural fear processing." *Proc Natl Acad Sci U S A* 109 (23):9203-8.

CHAPTER 5

1. Shapiro, I. M., E. J. Vresilovic, and M. V. Risbud. 2012. "Is the spinal motion segment a diarthrodial polyaxial joint: what a nice nucleus like you doing in a joint like this?" *Bone* 50 (3):771-6.

2. Johannaber, K. and F. A. Fathallah. 2012. "Spinal disc hydration status during simulated stooped posture." *Work* (41) Suppl 1:2384-6.

3. Race, A., N. D. Broom, and P. Robertson. 2000. "Effect of Loading Rate and Hydration on the Mechanical Properties of the Disc." *Spine (Phila Pa 1976)* 25 (6):662-9.

4. Dimitriadis, A., F. Smith, A. F. Mavrogenis, M. H. Pope, P. J. Papagelopoulos, A. Karantanas, A. Hadjipavlou, and P. Katonis. 2012. "Effect of two sitting postures on lumbar sagittal alignment and intervertebral discs in runners." *Radiol Med* 117 (4):654-68.

5. Holm, S., and A. Nachemson. 1983. "Variations in the nutrition of the canine intervertebral disc induced by motion." *Spine (Phila Pa 1976)* 8 (8):866-74.

6. Danneels, L. A., P. L. Coorevits, A. M. Cools, G. G. Vanderstraeten, D. C. Cambier, E. E. Witvrouw, and C. H. De. 2002. "Differences in electromyographic activity in the multifidus muscle and the iliocostalis lumborum between healthy subjects and patients with sub-acute and chronic low back pain." *Eur Spine J* 11 (1):13-9.

7. Carter, D. R. 2000. "Mechanobiology in rehabilitation science." *J Rehabil Res Dev* 37 (2):vii-viii.

8. Luike, M., S. Solovieva, A. Lamminen, K. Luoma, P. Leino-Arias, R. Luukkonen, and H. Riihimäki. 2005. "Disc degeneration of the lumbar spine in relation to overweight." *Int J Obes (Lond)* 29 (8):903-8.

9. Urban, J. P., S. Smith, and J. C. Fairbank. 2004. "Nutrition of the intervertebral disc." *Spine (Phila Pa 1976)* 29 (23):2700-9.

10. Parker-Pope, Tara. "Patients Hit the Weights in New Back-Pain Cure." *Wall Street Journal*, November 12, 2002. http://www.wsj.com/articles/SB1037053501459261588.

11. Holm, S., and A. Nachemson, 866-74.

12. Hansraj, K. K. 2014. "Assessment of stresses in the cervical spine caused by posture and position of the head." *Surg Technol Int* 25:277-9.

13. Bever, Lindsey. "'Text neck' is becoming an 'epidemic' that could wreck your spine." *The Washington Post*, November 20, 2014. http://www.washington-post.com/news/morning-mix/wp/2014/11/20/text-neck-is-becoming-an-epidemic-and-could-wreck-your-spine/.

14. Hansraj, K. K., 277-9.

15. Jensen, M. C., M. N. Brant-Zawadzki, N. Obuchowski, M. T. Modic, D. Malkasian, and J. S. Ross. 1994. "Magnetic resonance imaging of the lumbar spine in people without back pain." *N Engl J Med* 331 (2):69-73.

16. Lee, J. "Rethinking spine care." *Modern Healthcare*, March 22, 2014. http://www.modernhealthcare.com/article/20140322/MAGAZINE/303229985.

17. Ibid.

18. Chou, R., J. Baisden, E. J. Carragee, D. K. Resnick, W. O. Shaffer, and J. D. Loeser. 2009. "Surgery for low back pain: a review of the evidence for an American Pain Society Clinical Practice Guideline." *Spine (Phila Pa 1976)* 34 (10):1094-109.

CHAPTER 6

1. Daru, K. R. 1989. "Computer simulation and static analysis of the human head, neck and upper torso." Arizona State University.

2. Winters J. M. and J. D. Peles. 1990. "Neck muscle activity and 3-D head kinematics during quasi-static and dynamic tracking movements." In *Multiple Muscle Systems: Biomechanics and Movement Organization*, edited by Woo, S. L.-Y. and J. M. Winters, New York: Springer-Verlad.

3. Harris, William. "Will the Leaning Tower of Pisa ever fall?" Accessed February 20, 2015. http://science.howstuffworks.com/engineering/structural/will-leaning-tower-of-pisa-fall.htm.

4. Wilke, H. J., P. Neef, M. Caimi, T. Hoogland, and L. E. Claes. 1999. "New in vivo measurements of pressures in the intervertebral disc in daily life." *Spine (Phila Pa 1976)* 24 (8):755-62.

5. Nachemson, A. L. 1981. "Disc pressure measurements." *Spine (Phila Pa 1976)* 6 (1):93-7.

6. Parker-Pope, Tara. "Patients Hit the Weights in New Back-Pain Cure." *Wall Street Journal*, November 12, 2002. http://www.wsj.com/articles/ SB1037053501459261588.

7. Melone, Linda. "4 Big Benefits From Strength Training." *Arthritis Foundation*, Accessed April 7, 2014. http://www.arthritistoday.org/about-arthritis/ types-of-arthritis/rheumatoid-arthritis/daily-life/stay-ing-active/strength-training-benefits.php.

8. Andrews, M. A. W. 2003. "How does exercise make your muscles stronger?" *Scientific American.* http:// www.scientificamerican.com/article/how-does-ex-ercise-make-yo/.

9. Rainville, J., C. Hartigan, E. Martinez, J. Limke, C. Jouve, and M. Finno. 2004. "Exercise as a treatment for chronic low back pain." *Spine J* 4 (1):106-15.

CHAPTER 7

1. Lally, P., C. H. M. van Jaarsveld, H. W. W. Potts, and J. Wardle. 2010. "How are habits formed: Modeling habit formation in the real world." *Eur J Soc Psychol* 40 (6):998-1009.

2. Ibid.

3. Wansink, B., J. E. Painter, and J. North. 2005. "Bottom-less bowls: why visual cues of portion size may influence intake." *Obes Res* 13:93-100.

4. Milne, S., S. Orbell, and P. Sheeran. 2002. "Combining motivational and volitional interventions to promote exercise participation: protection motivation theory and implementation intentions." *Br J Health Psychol* 7 (Pt 2):163-84.

5. Moore, Monique and Wendy Nilsen. "6 Empirically-supported Tips for Forming Positive Habits." *Defense Centers of Excellence.* Accessed March 7, 2015. http://www.dcoe.mil/libraries/documents/6_empirically- supported_tips_for_forming_positive_habits.pdf.

6. Duhigg, C. 2012. *The Power of Habit: Why We Do What We Do in Life and in Business.* New York: Random House, Inc.: 76-8, 144-53.

7. Ibid.

8. Lally, P., C. H. M. van Jaarsveld, H. W. W. Potts, and J. Wardle, 998-1009.

9. Prochaska, James O., John Norcross, and Carlo DiClemente. 2009. *Changing for Good: A Revolutionary Six-Stage Program for Overcoming Bad Habits and Moving Your Life Positively Forward.* New York: William Morrow Paperbacks: 211.

10. Lally, P., C. H. M. van Jaarsveld, H. W. W. Potts, and J. Wardle, 998-1009.

11. Neal, David T., Wendy Wood, and Jeffrey M. Quinn. 2006. "Habits—A Repeat Performance." *Current Directions in Psychological Science* 15 (4):198-202.

12. Prochaska, James O., John Norcross, and Carlo DiClemente: 141-44, 195-98.

13. Park, Madison. 2012. "Rick Warren and church tackle obesity." *CNN*. Accessed August 9, 2015. http://edition.cnn.com/2012/01/24/health/saddleback-warren-diet/.

14. Townsend, S. S. M., H. S. Kim, and B. Mesquita. 2014. "Are you feeling what I'm feeling? Emotional similarity buffers stress." *Social Psychological and Personality Science* 5 (5):526-533.

15. Uchino, Bert N. 2004. *Social Support and Physical Health: Understanding the Health Consequences of Relationships, Current Perspectives in Psychology.* New Haven: Yale University Press: 80-93.

16. Reynolds, Gretchen. 2012. "The 'Love' Hormone as Sports Enhancer." *The New York Times*. Accessed June 24, 2015. http://well.blogs.nytimes.com/2012/11/21/the-love-hormone-as-sports-enhancer/?_r=2.

CHAPTER 8

1. Porter, Michael E. and Thomas H. Lee. 2013. "The Strategy that Will Fix Health Care." *Harvard Business Review.* https://hbr.org/2013/10/the-strategy-that-will-fix-health-care.

2. Ibid.

ABOUT THE AUTHOR

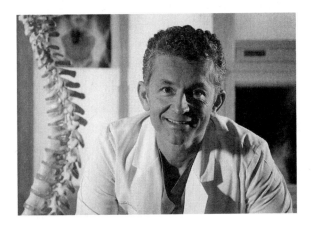

Kamshad Raiszadeh, MD, is a clinical instructor at the University of California, San Diego, founder/director of the Spine Institute of San Diego, and chief medical officer and co-founder of SpineZone Medical Fitness. He is a board-certified, fellowship-trained spine surgeon, member of the Scoliosis Research Society, and expert in minimally invasive surgery with an active surgical practice in San Diego, CA. He believes that we each deserve a life of vitality and full function—and that we can create it for ourselves by actively engaging in our recovery from chronic back pain.

Dr. Raiszadeh has an unusual perspective for a spine surgeon. Early on in his career, he realized that for most chronic back and neck pain patients, surgery is rarely the best solution. Convinced that there must be a better way, he and his team set about designing, developing, and perfecting a program that utilizes the best science in back care administered by different spinal specialists to empower patients. The team uses a high-tech, high-touch method to closely monitor patients and guide them through the program.

Over the past 10 years, his group has grown Spine-Zone into a highly successful, non-operative, multi-specialty clinic that has been shown to decrease or eliminate the need for surgery, injections, and addictive opioids. Besides its emphasis on strengthening weakened core muscles, SpineZone has used education, self-empowerment, and psychological health techniques to help close to 30,000 patients enjoy full and lasting recoveries.